3

TO LOSE

IN 3 WEEKS

Judith Wills is one of Britain's best-known and most knowledgeable slimming and nutrition experts and the author of *The Diet Bible*. Former editor of *Slimmer* magazine, she has also made three bestselling health videos and is an acclaimed cookery writer. Judith bases her writing on sound scientific principles and up-to-date research. Her nutritional advice follows World Health Organisation and Department of Health guidelines and her life as a working mother gives her insight into the problems the average person faces when they try to adopt healthy habits.

Also by Judith Wills:

Slim for Life

Fat Attack

Size 12 in 21 Days

Take Off Ten Years in Ten Weeks

The Bodysense Diet

100 Favourite Slim and Healthy Recipes

Slim and Healthy Vegetarian

The Omega Diet

The Food Bible

The Diet Bible

headline

3 WAYS
TO LOSE HALF A STONE
IN 3 WEEKS

Judith Wills

Fitness consultant Sarah McClurey

<u>headline</u>

First published as *6 Ways to Lose a Stone in 6 Weeks* in 1999
by HEADLINE BOOK PUBLISHING

First published in paperback in 2000
by HEADLINE BOOK PUBLISHING

This edition produced specially for Zest in 2002

ISBN 0 7553 1242 2

Designed by Isobel Gillan

Printed and bound in Great Britain by
Mackays of Chatham, Plc, Chatham, Kent

HEADLINE BOOK PUBLISHING
A division of the Hodder Headline Group
338 Euston Road
London NW1 3BH

www.headline.co.uk
www.hodderheadline.com

Contents

Introduction vi

3 ways to lose half a stone – which one is right for you? viii

The Detox and Energise Plan 1

The Healthy Fast Food Plan 24

The Sweet-tooth Plan 51

The 'E' Word 79

introduction

What is it about half a stone? Those seven little pounds are so easy to gain and yet can be so difficult to lose. Whether it's the first half stone to kickstart a bigger weight loss plan or the last few pounds to get you to your ideal weight, half a stone is a milestone in any weight loss regime. If you want to lose seven pounds but just can't seem to find the right eating plan or enough motivation to do it, this is the book for you.

If your attempts to lose weight have failed in the past, it's probably because you gave up all the foods you love then inevitably succumbed to your cravings within a few days. In *Three Ways to Lose Half a Stone in Three Weeks* you've got the choice of three eating plans so you can choose the one most suited to you and the foods you like. Yes, you can enjoy food and still lose weight!

If you feel in need of a cleansing, reviving diet, then the Detox and Energise Plan is the one for you. Over three weeks your tastebuds will be enlivened with quality, natural foods with a high emphasis on fruits, vegetables and raw foods.

Or if you want to eat healthily but have little time to spare, the Healthy Fast Food Plan may be just what you need. It majors on all the foods that are quick and easy to prepare and yet also good for you. You can eat takeaways and drink some alcohol as part of this healthy plan.

And if you want to lose weight but can't live without a regular daily fix of chocolate, biscuits, puddings or sugar in your coffee, you'll love the Sweet-tooth Plan. Even better, it shows you how to manage that sweet tooth, rather than *it* managing *you*.

Whichever one you pick, if you follow the plan we GUARANTEE it WILL work and in three weeks you'll have lost that half a stone.

The two most important things to remember are to do regular exercise along with the diet, and to get organised, food-wise, at the start of every week.

So what are you waiting for . . . start now and get ready for a fabulous new you!

Judith Wills

3 ways to lose half a stone - which one is right for you?

The next 3 chapters offer three different slimming programmes to help you lose half a stone.

They are the Detox and Energise Plan, The Healthy Fast Food Plan and the Sweet-tooth plan. If you are not sure which of the plans is right for you at this time, use the following questionnaire to help you decide. Simply answer the three sets of questions and add up your 'yes' answers for each set, then see for which set you have most often answered 'yes'. This then is probably your favoured plan.

Detox and Energise

	Yes	No
Do you feel below par, lacking in energy, run down?	☐	☐
Do you feel that your diet is unhealthy, with too many high-fat, high-sugar, high-salt and processed products?	☐	☐
Do you feel like making a new beginning?	☐	☐
Will your lifestyle allow you to eat plenty of fresh food *or* are you prepared to change your lifestyle and place more emphasis on healthy diet?	☐	☐
Are you happy to eat little meat and animal produce?	☐	☐
Do you tend to get digestive problems, perhaps including bloating, constipation, fluid retention?	☐	☐
Is good health one of your main motivators for slimming?	☐	☐
Do you enjoy the idea of simplicity and minimalism within your diet?	☐	☐

Healthy Fast Food

	Yes	No
Do you lead a very busy lifestyle which you feel unable to change?	☐	☐
Do you rely a lot on convenience meals and fast food?	☐	☐
Do you resent time spent cooking?	☐	☐
Have you found on any previous attempts to lose weight that you had to give up because healthy reduced-calorie food seemed too time-consuming?	☐	☐
Are you happy to eat 'little and often'?	☐	☐
Do you live alone, or, at least, require meals just for yourself?	☐	☐
Are you happy to pay a little extra for healthy fast food?	☐	☐
Do you enjoy a wide variety of foods?	☐	☐

Sweet-tooth

	Yes	No
Do you like chocolate and/or confectionery?	☐	☐
Do you like puddings and desserts?	☐	☐
Do you like biscuits, cakes and other sweet snacks?	☐	☐
Do you like the idea of incorporating sweet foods into a healthy slimming plan?	☐	☐
Would you like to learn how to control the urge to overindulge in sweet foods?	☐	☐
Do you like a wide variety of other foods?	☐	☐
Would you call yourself an organised person?	☐	☐
Are you prepared to accept that you can't lose weight steadily unless you are prepared to modify your diet to include sweet foods in reasonable but not excessive quantities?	☐	☐

chapter one

the detox and energise plan

Often when you decide you want to lose weight, you also embark on a fitness regime – because you want not only to look better but also to feel better. It makes sense, then, to use this time when your motivation levels are so high to treat yourself to a diet that will not only help you lose pounds, but also help you to feel more energised, more healthy.

That is the basis of my Detox and Energise programme.

Detoxing

I used to think that there was no such thing as the detox effect and that products and diets claiming to help you to detox were just a con. However, having done a lot of research on the subject, I have come to the conclusion that a carefully thought-out programme can, indeed, detox your system, re-educate your palate and re-energise your body.

To detox means to rid your body of toxins (poisons). The first questions I set out to answer were – do our bodies really carry toxins? If so, do we need help in getting rid of these? And can diet possibly do such a thing?

The answers to these three questions seem to be Yes, usually; Yes, usually; and Yes, it can.

The human body can contain toxins which have arrived in various ways: in our food and drink (pesticide and herbicide residues, hormone and antibiotic residues, artificial additives of many kinds, and alcohol, for example); because of a modern lifestyle (high levels of toxic chemicals such as carbon monoxide in the atmosphere or aluminium in pans or chemicals in food wrap, and tobacco smoke, for example); because of illness or perceived illness (viruses and bacteria are toxins, and even the 'cures' may be toxic if taken over long periods, including vitamin and mineral supplements, paracetamol and similar remedies).

If you are young, fit, healthy and stress free, your body's own defence and filter system (the lymph glands, liver and kidneys) may be able to deal with these toxins on its own, helping to remove them from the body in waste matter, urine, sweat and on the breath. But frequent ailments, feeling less than wonderful, perhaps with bloating and mildly enlarged glands around the body (the neck is a typical site for enlarged glands), all indicate that your body's toxin disposal system may need some help.

This can be done simply in three ways:
- by choosing a diet as low in probable sources of toxins as possible;
- by choosing foods, drinks and supplements which will actively aid the elimination of toxins; and
- by suitable exercise and a healthy lifestyle.

Energising

A detox regime marries very well with a revitalising, energising diet. Foods that may help your energy levels are fruits (high in natural sugars, vitamin C and phytochemicals – the 'active X factor' ingredients in natural foods that experts are now beginning to realise may hold an important key to good health and long life); vegetables (also high in vitamin C and phytochemicals as well as important minerals such as iron, selenium and calcium); complex carbohydrates (found in starchy foods such as rice and other grains, and potatoes), and essential fats (found in large quantities in plant, seed and nut oils, seeds and nuts and oily fish).

A diet combining all these foods will also be high in the anti-oxidants vitamins A, C and E and selenium. Anti-oxidants help to neutralise 'free radicals' in the body – substances which are produced in the body as a normal by-product of metabolism, but which may be produced in excess when the body is under stress or subject to pollution. It is thought that these free radicals are responsible for the human ageing process and in excess may be linked with all kinds of illnesses including cancers and arterial disease.

Weight loss

Because the Detox and Energise Plan is so natural and so naturally low in saturated fats and added sugars, most people will find that they lose weight very easily on it. There is also virtually no measuring of food, which is another bonus.

How the plan works

Lots of detox programmes last for only two or three days and throw you straight in at the deep end – going directly from your normal eating habits to a virtual fast. A short, sharp detox like that isn't ideal.

For one thing it is always best to prepare your body – and your mind – for a detox programme by going into it gradually. Your digestive system needs to adjust over a period of a week or two otherwise you could suffer from indigestion, wind and perhaps a loose bowel. And for another thing, it takes more than a couple of days for the detoxification to work. Toxins that the lymph, liver and kidneys have not been able to deal with are stored in body fat and, as we've seen, you can't lose more than a tiny amount of body fat in a day or two.

Lastly, a fast or near-fast will nearly always result in your feeling lethargic and perhaps dizzy with a headache and will also result in unnecessary loss of lean body tissue from muscle and organs.

There is no need to fast in order to detox. My gradual plan helps to eliminate these symptoms and should actually help to energise you.

What you are going to do, then, is gradually to cut down – or in some cases cut out – the dietary items that may have been contributing to a toxic state, while gradually building up the 'good' items.

Exercise

For the detox to work at optimum level, you need to take regular moderate exercise outdoors. This is to help stimulate your lymph glands to work efficiently and is particularly important if you have been prone to fluid retention and bloating. Have you ever noticed how you need to 'go to the loo' when you come in from a brisk walk, cycle ride, swim or whatever? That is because the exercise has stimulated the lymph system. Your blood flow is also improved which helps in the detox process. You will have 'worked up a sweat', eliminating toxins that way. And lastly you should have filled your lungs with oxygen-rich air, helping to remove toxins through the breath.

Lifestyle

As I have said, some toxins are present because of a poor lifestyle. While following the Detox and Energise Plan, you should not smoke tobacco, drink alcohol or take drugs of any kind other than mandatory ones prescribed by your doctor. (If you have any particular medical conditions you should ask your doctor if this plan is suitable for you to follow.) You should also avoid vitamin and mineral supplements unless completely natural (lots of supplements are artificially manufactured and may themselves contain possible toxins or allergens).

You should get plenty of sleep, rest and relaxation and try to reduce stress levels. You should sleep with an open window in a cool room. And you should make time for yourself and your diet.

Organic food

Ideally you should eat and drink nothing but organic produce while on the detox. This will be guaranteed free from agro-chemicals and additives. All of our basic food – fruit, vegetables, milk, meat, eggs and so on – may contain traces of residues such as pesticides, herbicides and fungicides.

All major supermarkets now have a wide range of organic produce on offer. You can also join a box scheme, where organic produce is delivered to your door weekly (for information telephone the Soil Association on 0117 929 0661). You can also look in the small ad columns of Sunday papers, food magazines and so on for small companies who specialise in various types of organic produce by mail order – these are particularly good for meat, fish and cheese. Yes, organic food is more expensive than mass-produced non-organic food, but I have found that most people beginning a plan such as this one will actually find that they save money on their grocery bill over the three weeks. That is because 'added value' high-cost foods – processed, ready to eat, take-aways, and so on – are not featured, and also because the overall calorie consumption is reduced. What you save on all the junk and unnecessary food you spend on gorgeous, wholesome, better-tasting food that really is good for you! Don't begrudge it.

Here is a list of items that you should seek out in their organic form:

- Poultry
- Fish
- Eggs
- Dairy produce
- Fruit
- Vegetables
- Pulses
- Bread
- Grains, including rice, breakfast cereals, etc.

Wholefoods

During the programme, all your foods should be 'whole' – in other words, not refined. Avoid white bread, white rice, white pasta, refined sugar, anything other than whole-grain breakfast cereals and so on. Wholefoods contain more vital vitamins such as the B-group, more fibre for a healthy digestive system and more of some other trace elements.

Pulses can be canned in water, but not in brine. Rinse and drain well before use.

Where to obtain the more unusual detox plants, herbs, etc.

You will find some fairly unusual plants, herbs, roots, etc. listed below, all of which can help your body to eliminate toxins. You will not find many of them in your local supermarket and you may need either to visit a well-stocked health-food shop, which should keep organic dried versions of the items mentioned, or else send off for a mail order catalogue to a reputable company, such as Neal's Yard Remedies (telephone 0161 831 7875 for details).

If you live in the country, you may also be able to pick some of the plants yourself – even from your own garden! Who hasn't got dandelion and nettles growing somewhere near by, for example? If you are going to try seeking some of the other plants, arm yourself with a good book on wild food (such as Richard Mabey's *Food For Free*) so that you don't end up picking the wrong thing and poisoning yourself – **NOT** the idea of this plan at all! Wash all plants thoroughly and avoid using plants that have been growing close to a road. Page 19 explains how to make your own herbal teas and decoctions. It is very easy.

Getting organised

Before you begin, sort out your store-cupboard, refrigerator, etc., and chuck out things that you won't want to be eating, to make room for the items that you will.

Make a shopping list to take you through at least the first week, and thereafter shop regularly for what you need.

Store your food in cool and dark conditions, properly wrapped, to retain maximum vitamins C and B, and use it regularly.

Because you will be 'de-cluttering' your eating life (this plan is ideal for minimalists) you should in the long run save time on your food.

Foods and drinks to help your detox

These pages are a quick reference to good sources of a variety of nutrients and plant chemicals which will aid your Detox and Energise Plan. Over the weeks ahead they will come to form a large part of your diet.

- *Vitamin C* A powerful anti-oxidant which helps maintain healthy skin, gums, eyes. Also important for absorption of iron. Excellent sources – blackcurrants, kiwi fruit, rosehips, citrus fruits, sweet peppers, broccoli, sprouts, parsley, strawberries, mango, guava, melon, tomatoes, leafy greens, fresh chilli peppers. Most fresh and frozen fruits and vegetables contain some vitamin C; canned contain very little and should be avoided. Storage, light and heat deplete foods of their vitamin C content.
- *Vitamin E* Another anti-oxidant vital for healthy soft skin, its anti-ageing properties, and its ability to bolster the body's immune system. Excellent sources – wheatgerm oil, sunflower oil and seeds, safflower oil, hazelnuts, sun-dried tomatoes, almonds, corn oil, groundnut oil, pine nuts, Brazil nuts, sweet potato, other nuts (fresh, not salted). Store E-rich oily foods in cool dark conditions and use quickly – they can go rancid and oxidise.
- *Vitamin B group* Six individual vitamins that work together to help the body maintain metabolic processes, energy levels and in various other tasks. Good sources – whole grains, fish, eggs, poultry, lean pork, yeast extract, but also present in a wide variety of healthy foods and so a varied diet is essential.
- *Beta-carotene* Anti-oxidant which helps boost the immune system and mop up surplus free radicals. Excellent sources – carrots, sweet potato, dark leafy greens, sweet peppers, chilli peppers, mango,

orange-fleshed squash, orange-fleshed melon, tomatoes, broccoli.

- **Selenium** Anti-oxidant mineral which works with vitamin E. Strong likelihood of shortage in the diet. Excellent sources – Brazil nuts. Good sources – green or brown lentils, canned or fresh tuna, mullet, squid, sardines, sunflower seeds, white fish, wholemeal bread, salmon, walnuts, lean pork.

- **Zinc** Another mineral important to help keep the immune system and liver healthy and eliminate toxins. Good sources – wheatgerm, seeds, nuts, All-Bran, shellfish, lean red meat, Quorn.

- **Iron** Carries oxygen from the lungs through the body, helps healing and the immune system. Lack of iron (fairly common in females) can cause lethargy and lack of energy. Excellent low saturated-fat sources of iron – ground ginger, seaweed, All-Bran, green or brown lentils, sesame and pumpkin seeds, soya beans, Weetabix, dried peaches and apricots, bulghar wheat, pot barley, brown rice, dark leafy greens, broccoli. Lean red meat and eggs are a good source of easily absorbed iron and are allowed in the first two weeks of the diet but contain a moderate amount of saturated fat.

- **Essential fats** Two types of polyunsaturated fat which are important for the smooth and efficient functioning of the body including weight control. May also help the immune system and to maintain energy levels. Essential fats are found in excellent quantities in seed and nut oils as well as in seeds and nuts themselves. Several other plant foods and fish contain reasonable amounts of one or other of the two essential fatty acids.

- **Fibre** Adequate fibre in the diet is important on this plan to help the speedy passage of food through the gut, thus helping the elimination process. It will also help prevent hunger. Fibre is found only in plant foods. Excellent sources are pulses, pot barley, All-Bran, whole grains, peas and beans, parsnips, sprouts, dried apricots, figs and prunes, leafy green vegetables. All unrefined plant foods contain some fibre. Refined cereals contain very little.

- **Diuretics** Certain plants can help the body eliminate fluid in the urine quickly – important if you are prone to fluid retention and bloating. Some of these are dandelion, nettles, parsley, tarragon, dock root, cucumber, onions and apples.

- **Plants to aid liver function** Poor liver and gallbladder function can slow down the elimination of toxins. Help your liver cope with the aid of dandelion root, marigold, parsley, burdock leaves or root, peppermint leaves, dock root, apples, cucumber, onions, artichoke hearts, beetroot juice and olive oil. A supplement of milk thistle can also be taken, available from health food shops or by mail order.
- **Plants to aid lymph function** Stimulate your lymph system into working well with the help of angelica, lovage, marigold, rosemary, dock, ginger, cayenne, oregano.
- **Laxatives** Natural laxatives can be incorporated into the diet to help eliminate waste matter. These are rhubarb, prunes, licorice, olive oil, burdock, dock, and aloe vera juice. All the high-fibre foods will also help to prevent constipation.
- **Heating foods** Elimination through perspiration can be increased by including 'heating' foods in the diet. These are most spices, particularly mustard and chillies; garlic, onions, green tea, rosemary and thyme.

Unlimiteds

- **Foods** All organic fresh and frozen green vegetables and salad items.
- **Condiments** Fresh herbs or dried herbs and spices, lemon juice, unsalted tomato purée, passata, good quality wine vinegar, unsalted vegetable stock/cubes.
- **Drinks** Water, mineral water, organic herbal teas, decoctions and infusions (see page 19); unsweetened fruit teas, green tea; fresh home-made fruit juices diluted with water; fresh home-made vegetable juices (**NOTE** limit carrot juice to one glass a day).

Remember to drink four pints of fluid a day.

WEEK ONE

Goals for the week

Eat/drink more

- Fresh fruits, especially any of those listed on pages 7–9 which are rich in vitamin C or beta-carotene, or apples. Aim for three portions a day. This is easy to do if you have fruit every day at breakfast, with/as one snack a day and at either lunchtime or after your evening meal.
- Leafy green vegetables. Aim for a minimum of one portion a day.
- Water or similar. Four pints a day is ideal. Herbal teas count towards your water intake. This week try dandelion-root tea to help liver function (see recipe page 19) or try any of the herbs mentioned in the list on page 9.

Cut down on

- Added salt. Stop adding salt to food on your plate and cut down on the amount you add in cooking.
- Fat. Choose lean meats and give yourself smaller portions than usual, remove all visible fat off food, cut by half the fat you put on bread, etc., skim all fat off pan juices when roasting before making gravy/sauce, and try to choose lower-fat cheeses such as Brie, Camembert, Edam, feta, light cream cheese, half-fat Cheddar, Halloumi and cottage cheese rather than higher-fat ones like Cheddar, Stilton, cream cheese and Cambazola.
- Caffeine. Cut down on the amount of tea and/or coffee that you drink. Make it weaker. (Choose herbal drinks instead, see below and page 19.) Cut down on the amount of chocolate you eat and choose good quality plain organic chocolate (e.g. Green and Black's).
- Highly processed foods. Try to avoid packet and canned foods, especially those with lots of E numbers (read the ingredients label), such as soups, sauce mixes, snack foods, instant desserts.

Avoid

- Added sugar. Don't add sugar to cereals, drinks, etc. Try to do without artificial sweetener. If necessary, cut down the amount of sugar you use gradually this week, day by day.
- Sweet, highly refined foods. Avoid cakes, packet biscuits, sugary desserts, sweet pastries, baked goods and all confectionery except good chocolate.
- All pastry.
- Take-away meals and ready-to-heat meals.
- Cola and all other carbonated commercial drinks.
- Percolated coffee and cafetière coffee.
- All milk except skimmed milk or soya milk.

Notes

- Don't forget your unlimited items listed on page 9.
- Have a Breakfast, Lunch, Evening Meal plus two healthy Snacks and plenty to drink every day. Do try to make your own fresh fruit and vegetable juices. Any juices mentioned in the meal suggestions are ideas only – feel free to juice whenever you like.
- Try to buy everything organic, or at least free range.
- Eat enough to satisfy hunger but no more.
- Each week the meal suggestions are samples only; try to add a few ideas of your own that fit in with the guidelines above and include plenty of unlimited items.

BREAKFASTS

- Portion vitamin C- and/or fibre-rich fruit; All-Bran; natural bio yogurt.
- Brown toast with a scraping of butter; low-sugar jam; natural bio yogurt; fresh citrus juice.
- 'No added sugar or salt' muesli, with 1 banana and skimmed milk to cover.
- Boiled egg; 1 slice wholewheat toast with a scraping of butter; 1 portion vitamin C- and/or fibre-rich fruit.

LUNCHES

- Wholewheat sandwich filled with Brie and sliced tomato; 1 portion fruit of choice; 1 slice malt loaf.
- Low-salt baked beans on toast; vitamin C-rich fruit; 1 apple.
- Lean cooked chicken with tomato, green pepper and Cos salad; Ryvitas; 1 fruit-flavoured fromage frais; 1 portion fruit of choice.
- Eggs on brown toast with a scraping of butter; 1 orange; 1 Greek yogurt.
- Wholewheat pasta, avocado and tomato salad; 1 small portion grilled Halloumi cheese; beetroot or apple juice.

EVENING MEALS

- Small lean steak; new potatoes; leafy greens; peas; apricot juice.
- Baked white fish; oven chips; peas; tomato salad.
- Brown rice topped with selection of grilled Mediterranean vegetables and garnished with either small amount of grated Parmesan cheese or poached egg; fresh fruit juice.
- Baked potato; baked beans or home-made chilli con carne; large mixed salad.
- Roast or grilled chicken or turkey (skin removed) with lemon and tarragon; new potatoes; broccoli; puréed parsnips; carrots; skimmed pan juices.

SNACKS

- Fresh fruit.
- Staffordshire oatcake and hummus.
- Small piece plain organic chocolate or cheese and apple.
- Bio yogurt with fruit purée.

WEEK **TWO**

Goals for the week

Eat more

All items as Week 1 plus:

- Salad, including tomatoes, onions, cucumber, dark lettuce leaves, rocket, watercress, spinach.
- Fresh herbs – see page 9.
- Fish, both white and oily. Mackerel, herring, salmon, trout, sardines and tuna are oily.
- Dried fruits – go for apricots, peaches, prunes and figs rather than sultanas, raisins and currants.

Try to cut down on

- High salt foods. These include many cheeses, processed foods, soy sauce.
- Added salt. Cut again the amount you use in cooking.
- Chocolate. Cut down again on the amount of chocolate you eat; limit to one square a day.
- All animal flesh. Limit to twice in the week.
- Bread and wheat-based products such as crackers. Limit bread to one slice a day.

Avoid

All items as Week 1 plus:

- Refined flour, cereals and grains. That includes all bread except wholemeal, breakfast cereals such as cornflakes, crisped rice, white pasta, white rice.
- All highly processed packet foods and all canned foods except pulses canned in water and tomatoes.
- Black tea, coffee, squashes.

- Full-fat cheese, including Cheddar, Stilton, soft blue cheeses, cream cheese.

Notes

As Week 1.

BREAKFASTS

- Fresh berry fruits; natural low-fat bio yogurt; oat flakes.
- Fruit Compôte (see recipe page 23); natural 8 per cent fat fromage frais; muesli; fresh fruit juice.
- Fresh citrus fruit salad; Greek yogurt; grapenuts.
- Boiled egg; 2 rye crispbreads or 1 small slice whole rye bread; 1 orange.

LUNCHES

- Tabbouleh (see recipe page 21); 1 apple; 1 low-fat bio yogurt; beetroot juice.
- Brown rice and tuna (canned in water, drained) salad with watercress, hard-boiled egg, spinach and parsley; citrus juice.
- Salad of new potatoes with chopped mint, parsley, broad beans tossed in bio yogurt and lemon juice dressing; green salad; dried apricots.
- Salad of brown rice, chopped apple, chopped dried apricot, a little lean chicken; herb salad.
- Broccoli, Potato and Garlic Soup (see recipe page 20), ½ slice wholemeal bread; large mixed salad; 1 banana.

EVENING MEALS

- Poached salmon; new potatoes; large mixed salad or broccoli and peas.
- Lean chicken or turkey stir-fried in groundnut oil with selection of fresh vegetables; 1 small portion wholewheat noodles; Fruit Compôte (see recipe page 23).
- Sweet Potato Curry (see recipe page 22) and brown rice; portion vitamin C-rich fruit.
- White fish, grilled or baked; lemon; peas; green beans.
- Baked potato; natural 8 per cent fromage frais mixed with mustard; large mixed salad.

SNACKS

- Rye crispbread and hummus.
- Fresh fruit.
- Dried fruit.
- Low-fat bio yogurt and apple.

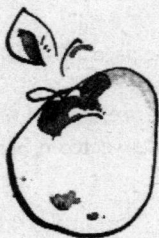

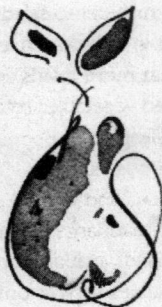

WEEK **THREE**

Goals for the week

Eat more

All items as previous weeks plus:

- Olive oil and other plant oils high in essential fatty acids.
- Fresh juices. Squeeze your own citrus juices. If you have a blender you can whizz all kinds of fruits and vegetables to make a 'complete' juice including the fruit/vegetable fibre. Juice extractors leave much of the fruit's goodness behind in the pulp.
- Herbal teas and herbs. The herbs listed on page 9 really do have a beneficial effect in helping your body to 'detox' – give some of them a try. One to two cups a day should help. Add fresh herbs to salads and sprinkle over vegetables. Garlic is another good herb to use regularly.
- Pulses. Now you've cut out meat, replace it in your diet with more high-protein, low-fat pulses such as kidney beans, soya beans (and tofu, which is made from soya), butter beans, chickpeas and lentils. They can be mixed into salads, served as a vegetable or used to replace meat in dishes such as curries and casseroles.
- Raw foods. Eat more salads and nibble on raw vegetables during the day. Uncooked vegetables retain more of their vitamin C and can seem more filling.

Cut down on

- Grains of all kinds including breakfast cereals, rice, bulghar.
- Starchy vegetables such as potatoes, parsnips, sweetcorn, beetroot – have small portions only.

Avoid

All items as previous weeks plus:

- All bread and wheat products.
- Added salt – your tastebuds should have acclimatised by now.
- Chocolate.
- All dairy produce except skimmed milk and natural low-fat bio yogurt.
- Eggs.
- All meat, poultry and game.

Notes

As Week 1 plus:

- Calcium – It is important to get adequate calcium in the diet. One of our main sources is hard cheese and other dairy produce. As you are cutting right down on dairy products now it is vital to get calcium from other sources. Eat plenty of seeds, tofu, almonds, figs, Brazil nuts, dark green leafy vegetables and broccoli as well as unlimited low-fat bio yogurt and $\frac{1}{2}$ pint of skimmed milk *or* calcium-fortified soya milk daily. Milk can be blended with fruit for a morning shake.

BREAKFASTS

- Every day have a selection of fresh fruit and dried fruit with plenty of low-fat bio yogurt and a small handful of 'no added sugar or salt' muesli, plus a juice. Sprinkle with wheatgerm if liked.

LUNCHES

- Large fresh mixed salad including fresh herbs such as parsley and dark leaves such as rocket, spinach, lamb's lettuce; olive oil and vinegar dressing; small portion hummus made by blending cooked chickpeas with olive oil, lemon juice and black pepper; beetroot juice.
- Large fresh salad as above; sliced avocado and pine nuts mixed with 2 tablespoons cooked brown rice; apple juice.

- Fresh carrot and tomato soup (from chilled counter or home made); chopped parsley; fruit.
- Purée of butter beans (blended with a little olive oil and lemon juice) with selection of raw crudités; fruit.
- Broccoli soup (made by cooking broccoli in vegetable stock and puréeing); 1 banana.

EVENING MEALS

- Small baked potato; selection of steamed or baked Mediterranean vegetables including red peppers, onions, drizzled with olive or groundnut oil; peach juice.
- Stir-fried vegetables in sesame oil with cubed tofu, beansprouts, cabbage; carrots or similar; nuts or seeds; 1 slice melon.
- 2 tablespoons cooked brown rice with Sweet Potato Curry (see recipe page 22); 1 tablespoon low-fat bio yogurt; 1 orange.
- Baked trout with handful almonds; broccoli; spinach; fruit.
- Large mixed salad with olive oil dressing; sunflower seeds; 1 banana.

SNACKS

- Fruit.
- Dried fruit.
- Bio yogurt.
- Avocado purée with crudités.
- Skimmed milk and fruit blended into a shake with a little wheatgerm or wheatgerm oil if liked.

RECIPES FOR YOUR DETOX AND ENERGISE PLAN

INFUSIONS

An infusion is simply made as you would make ordinary tea. You make it from leaves or flowers of the plant, and it can also be called a tisane. Typical herbs that you might use to make an infusion are nettles, dandelion leaves, mint, lemon balm, marigold, rosemary or thyme.

The normal quantity of herb to water is one good tablespoon of fresh herb to half a pint of water. You can also use dried leaves or flowers to make an infusion, in which case one heaped teaspoonful is about the right amount.

Simply put the fresh or dried herb in a teapot or jug, pour on boiling water and leave to infuse for 5 minutes or so. Pour the tea into your cup or mug through a tea strainer and drink.

DECOCTIONS

Sometimes you may be using a part of the plant that is too tough or woody to make a good infusion – dandelion root or cinnamon sticks are two examples. In this case you need to decoct the herb. This means you chop it up and simmer it, uncovered, for about half an hour in water until enough of the 'active ingredient' of the herb has been released and the liquid is reduced by a third to a half, then strain and drink (or cool and refrigerate until needed). For one serving, one good tablespoon of chopped fresh plant or one good teaspoonful of dried plant to 250ml of water is about right.

BROCCOLI, POTATO AND GARLIC SOUP

Serves 2
175 calories and 6g fat per portion

1 dessertspoon sunflower seed oil
1 medium onion, chopped
1 large clove garlic, peeled and crushed
150g potato, peeled and chopped small
Black pepper
400ml organic low-salt vegetable stock
100g broccoli florets
1 dessertspoon chopped fresh mint
1 dessertspoon chopped fresh parsley
Low salt substitute (optional)
2 dessertspoons natural bio yogurt

Heat the oil in a saucepan and cook the onion over a medium low heat until softened, stirring occasionally. Add the garlic, potato, pepper and stock and bring to a simmer; cook for 15 minutes. Add the broccoli and simmer for another 5–7 minutes, then purée the soup in an electric blender. Return to the pan, stir in the mint, parsley and salt substitute if using, reheat, then serve with the yogurt swirled in.

NOTE *Home-made stock is easy to make – simply simmer carrot, onion, leek, celery in water with a small bouquet garni (or a few sprigs of thyme and parsley) for 30 minutes, then strain off the liquid.*

TABBOULEH

Serves 2
160 calories and 6.5g fat per portion

50g bulghar wheat
1 Little Gem lettuce or half a head of Cos
1 beef tomato, deseeded and chopped
4 spring onions, chopped
4cm chunk cucumber, chopped
1 handful fresh mint, chopped
1 handful fresh parsley, chopped
1 tablespoon olive oil
1 tablespoon lemon juice
Black pepper

Soak the bulghar wheat in just boiled water for 20 minutes and drain thoroughly. Slice the lettuce thinly lengthways and arrange on plates. In a bowl, mix together the bulghar wheat with the remaining ingredients and pile onto the lettuce.

SWEET POTATO CURRY

Serves 2
370 calories and 8g fat per portion

1 tablespoon groundnut oil
1 medium onion, thinly sliced
1 large or 2 small sweet potatoes (about 350g), peeled and
cut into cubes
1 clove garlic, peeled and crushed
½ teaspoon each of ground chilli, cumin, ginger, turmeric and
coriander seed
150g broccoli florets, parboiled
50g green lentils, simmered in water until tender and drained
200ml low-salt vegetable stock
100g baby leaf spinach or shredded spring greens
Black pepper
2 tablespoons natural whole-milk bio yogurt

Heat the oil in a large non-stick frying pan and sauté the onion and
sweet potato over a medium high heat, stirring frequently, until part
cooked and the potato is tinged golden. Add the garlic and spices and
stir for a minute or two, then add the broccoli, lentils and stock, bring
to a simmer, and cook, uncovered, for 10 minutes or until the sweet
potato and broccoli is almost cooked. Add the spinach (or greens),
black pepper and yogurt and stir, simmer for a minute to wilt the
greens, then serve. This is good served with chopped cucumber
tossed in a little low-fat bio yogurt plus finely chopped garlic, if liked.

NOTE *You can substitute some of the spinach or greens with fresh nettle
leaves if available.*

FRUIT COMPÔTE

Serves 4
110 calories and trace fat per portion

50g dried apricots
50g dried peaches
50g stoned dried prunes
50g dried figs
300ml fresh orange juice
Cinnamon stick
2 cloves
Lemon zest

Put the dried fruits in a saucepan, cover with the orange juice, adding water to cover as necessary. Tuck in the remaining ingredients and simmer, covered, for 30 minutes or until all the fruit is tender. Remove the cinnamon stick and cloves and serve warm or allow to cool. Store in an airtight container in the refrigerator for a maximum of 3 days.

NOTE *Fresh chopped fruit and/or nuts and seeds can be added to the compôte before serving.*

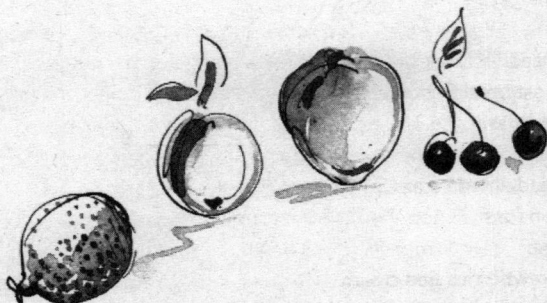

the healthy
fast food plan

So you like 'fast food' and you don't want to give it up. Or your lifestyle is so unavoidably busy, that even if you want to, you can't.

But you're overweight and you need to lose those pounds. So how can you reconcile snacking, convenience foods, and little time to spend in the kitchen with slimming?

It **CAN** be done – with a bit of know-how. And here's where to find that knowledge.

In fact, many foods that are quick and easy to prepare (or need no preparation at all) are, actually, healthy and good for you, and not as high in fat and calories as you might think. So to start with, just to cheer you up and put you in a positive frame of mind, here are my top 20 quick and easy foods that you can eat without guilt on your slimming plan:

- Bread
- Most breakfast cereals
- Bananas
- Pasta
- Ready-made soup
- Potatoes
- Eggs
- Strawberries and cream
- Dried fruit
- Steak

- Cheese
- Baked beans
- Rice
- Baked potatoes
- Pizza
- Curry
- Chinese meals
- Ready-made sandwiches
- Burgers
- Chips

There are also plenty of other foods which you probably already consider 'healthy' or 'slimming' but which you don't see as fast food that will fit in with your lifestyle – fruits, salads, vegetables, yogurts, pulses and so on. In this plan, I aim to show you that these are all legitimate and tasty contributors towards a quick and easy diet.

And then, of course, there are the items that many people eat too much of when they live on snacks and fast food – chocolate, biscuits, cakes, crisps, ready desserts, take-aways and fried foods. I am going to show you how to incorporate these tastes and textures into your life while you slim.

Why snacking isn't a sin!

People who haven't much time to spend on their diet often say to me that they feel guilty for snacking rather than having just three 'proper' meals a day.

In fact, there is no need to worry about eating more than three times a day – it is the **RIGHT** way to eat! All research shows that eating 'little and often' is healthier than the 'let's just have one meal a day' syndrome. Our digestive systems cope better with smaller, frequent meals; our metabolic rate burns slightly quicker on such a regime, and when we're trying to slim and cut down calories, hunger pangs are much easier to keep at bay if a plan that allows snacks is followed.

The thing to alter is, of course, the type of snacks you are eating. A recent survey found that chocolate bars and crisps are this country's two most favoured snacks. On pages 31–34 you will find a whole range of ideas for tasty, quick snacks with which you can replace these, and other favourite high-calorie snack foods.

The Healthy Fast Food Plan allows you plenty of scope for new snacks – and some of your old favourites!

Tips for healthy fast food shopping, cooking and eating

As any time management consultant will tell you, it is much quicker to be organised than to be disorganised, and that applies to your eating habits as much as anything else.

Many people who rely on fast food because they are so busy tend to grab what they can at the last minute; spend precious lunch breaks queuing for 'fast' food which turns out to be slower than making a packed lunch; spend valuable after-work time dashing out from home to the local supermarket or take-away because there's nothing in the refrigerator to eat – and so on.

Disorganised eating not only takes longer in the long run – it is also more likely to be the high-calorie eating that has helped you to put on half a stone or more. You really need to plan ahead for your food, however busy you are. One hour one day a week spent planning ahead and shopping for what you need really **WILL** save you time and many, many calories each and every week.

Getting organised

Once a week

- Take 10 minutes to plan your diet. Check through Week 1 of this programme and decide which meal options you're going to go for. You will see that every lunchtime, you have a choice of a Packed Lunch, a Home Lunch, or a Takeout. In the evenings you have a choice of a Make-Ahead Meal (quick-to-make recipes that will chill or freeze until needed), a Real Meal in Moments, or a Ready Meal. Decide in conjunction with your diary if necessary. (For example, plan to have a Make-Ahead evening meal or Ready Meal on a night when you will be late home, rather than a meal you cook from scratch, albeit a quick one.) As you do so, start a shopping list for any meals or snacks that you can prepare or will be eating at home. Have different sections for fruit, vegetables, meat and fish, canned goods, chilled goods, drinks, frozen food, etc. Also stock up on handy store-cupboard items which are a boon to busy people – pastas, rice, canned pulses, tomato sauces and passata, preserves, oriental sauces and so on. Keep all the sections in the order in which your favourite or most convenient store is laid out, which will save time when you shop.

- Take 30 minutes to shop. If you're shopping just for you it won't take more than this. When shopping, remember time is money and if time is your precious commodity rather than cash, go for labour-saving products such as ready-peeled fruit, ready-washed and bagged mixed salad, ready-diced meats, ready-peeled vegetables and so on. All these items will make you more inclined to eat healthily. Choose fresh produce with the latest 'sell-by' date so it will keep for longer at home.

- Take 5 minutes to put everything away tidily where it will be easy to find when you want it. Store fruits, vegetables and salad in the refrigerator. Most items will keep well for up to a week if correctly stored. If foods for the freezer, such as chicken portions and bread, can be split up into one-portion sizes, do so before freezing; they will be much more convenient this way when it is time to defrost – and there is less chance of you eating more than you need.

When you have a little spare time

- Take a few minutes to prepare your Make-Ahead evening meal(s), if chosen. Cover and put in refrigerator. If you can make double the quantity and freeze the other half, this will save you even more time.

Before bed

- If you are having a packed lunch, take a few minutes to make that before you go to bed and pop it in the refrigerator too.

Cooking tips

When preparing Make-Ahead Meals or Real Meals in Moments you can save a lot more time with these tips.

- If using the grill, put it on first to begin heating up while you do any necessary ingredient preparation.
- Always follow recipe instructions in the right order; they are designed to be time-saving.
- Get into the habit of using the microwave more for things like cooking chicken, fish, baked potatoes, quickly. It may be quicker to use hob and saucepan for vegetables.
- Many of the Meals in Moments and all the Make-Aheads can be frozen – so if you have time, make double the quantity and freeze the surplus.

Now read on for your instructions on following the Healthy Fast Food Plan.

Every day of every week on the diet, YOU PICK:

- *A Breakfast* (Some of which can be packed and eaten mid-morning if you prefer.)
- *A Lunch* Choose either a Packed Lunch, a Home Lunch (some hot, some cold), or Takeout option (food from sandwich bars, etc.). Try to limit a Takeout option to once or twice a week.
- *An Evening Meal* Choose either a Make-Ahead Meal (easy things you can cook in spare minutes and freeze or keep chilled until required); a Real Meal in Moments (suppers that can be on the table in between 10 and 20 minutes of starting the preparation);

or a Ready Meal (which is either a commercial chilled or frozen meal or a take-away). Try to limit Ready Meals to once or twice a week.

- *A Fruit Snack* Every day choose one portion of fruit of your choice. If choosing a banana, make it a small one. Occasionally you can have a 125ml glass of fruit juice instead; try to make this a chilled fresh juice rather than the long-life variety – dilute it with sparkling mineral water for a longer drink.

- *Milk Allowance* Have 250ml skimmed milk or 200ml semi-skimmed milk for use in tea and coffee or as a drink on its own. If not required, have 200ml low-fat natural bio yogurt instead – you need the calcium. Milk for breakfast cereals is on top of this allowance.

- *Snack Swaps* Every day choose 150 calories' worth of Snacks from the Snack Swaps on pages 31–4. Make these up as you like – e.g. six tiny 25-calorie snacks, one 100-calorie snack plus a 50, or whatever.

Unlimiteds

Every day you can have the following items in more or less unlimited quantity, though do try to go easy on artificially sweetened fizzy drinks and strong coffee.

- *Drinks* Tap water, mineral water, calorie-free drinks, weak tea or coffee (with milk from allowance, no sugar, use artificial sweeteners if necessary), herbal teas, green tea.

- *Food* Leafy green vegetables, green beans, runner beans, salad leaves, tomatoes, onion, courgettes, cucumber, celery, leeks, carrot, broccoli, cauliflower, aubergine, green peppers, yellow peppers – all raw or steamed, microwaved or boiled. Choose fresh or frozen and try to include as many of these as you can in your daily diet. They help fill you up and provide vitamins and minerals as well as fibre.

NOTE *Peas, broad beans, sweetcorn, red peppers and beetroot are higher in calories because they contain more sugar or starch and should be eaten in smaller quantities if choosing instead of the 'Unlimited' vegetables.*

- **Condiments** Fresh or dried herbs and spices, lemon juice, Worcestershire sauce, light soy sauce, tomato purée, passata, vinegar, low-fat stock cubes and garlic.

Week's Treats

Every week on the plan you can also have your Week's Treats. Have **ONE** of the following to use as and when you like during the week (with the exception of the alcohol, which should not be consumed all in one evening – spread it over 2–3 evenings at least). Keep strictly to the amounts of these treats given as they are high-calorie foods.

- **wine** I whole bottle of dry white or red wine, maximum alcohol by volume 12 per cent.
- **beer or lager or cider** Five half pints standard strength or ten half pints low alcohol.
- **crisps** Three bags standard crisps or similar (maximum weight 30g each).
- **chocolate** Two bars 4-finger KitKat or standard Dairy Milk or Flyte **OR** Five Halo Caramel or Nougat Bars (or five of any chocolate bar containing 100 calories or less).
- **desserts** Any five ready desserts calorie-counted on the pack at 100 or less per dessert (e.g. some of Boots Shapers range, many individual chocolate mousses).

SNACK SWAPS for Hungry Slimmers

Within the plan you are allowed up to 150 calories' worth of Snack Swaps every day. The Snack Swaps can be mixed and matched as you will to add up to that daily total. It might be an idea to carry round an insulated bag or small box containing your Snack Swaps, or keep them in the kitchen or your office desk, so that you always have a snack to hand when you want something to eat — fast.

If you feel like something **SWEET** instead of chocolates, sweets or ice cream, choose ...

For **25 calories** or less	For **50 calories** or less	For **100 calories** or less
3 ready-to-eat dried apricots	1 good handful Choco Cornflakes	2-biscuit pack Weight-Watchers Cookies
1 ready tub sugar-free jelly	1 Jaffa cake	Shape Greek Style Orange Yoghurt
1 Melba toast with low-sugar jam	1 sachet instant hot chocolate	1 Quaker Harvest Apple and Raisin Chewy Bar
1 ripe plum	1 French Toast with runny honey	1 Boots Shapers cereal bar, any variety
	1 dark rye Ryvita spread with 1 tsp Nutella	1 ready tub low-fat rice pudding
	1 peach, pear or orange	1 Häagen-Dazs frozen yogurt bar

If you feel like something **CRUNCHY** instead of high-fat crisps and other savoury snacks, choose ...

For **25 calories** or less	For **50 calories** or less	For **100 calories** or less
1 dark rye Ryvita	1 dark rye Ryvita with 1 tsp crunchy peanut butter	23g pack Butterkist popcorn
1 Slice a Rice	1 Pogens Crdisproll with Marmite	1 pack Boots Shapers Crisps or Crinkles, any variety
2 fresh carrots	1 Sharwood's ready cooked standard poppadom	1 pack Golden Lights Crisps
2 pieces Melba toast	15g dry All-Bran (try it – it is delicious!)	
	1 crisp apple	
	2 sesame Grissini sticks	

If you want something **SAVOURY** or **CHEESY** instead of greasy chips or a high-fat chunk of Cheddar, try ...

For **25 calories** or less	For **50 calories** or less	For **100 calories** or less
Spring onions dipped in any ready made salsa	Carrot sticks dipped in WeightWatchers Mayonnaise Dressing	100g cold cooked new potatoes sprinkled with sea salt
2 tablespoons cold baked beans	1 Babybel Light individual cheese	1 mini pitta with 40g ready tzatziki

1 slice Melba toast with 1 sachet 10-calorie soup

1 slice Melba toast with 1 tsp Philly Light or Marmite

1 slice Melba toast spread with WeightWatchers Mayonnaise Dressing and chopped onion

1 Cheestring

2 Grissini sticks with 50ml any tzatziki dip

1 dark rye Ryvita with 1 laughing cow cheese triangle

1 × 20g pack Go Ahead Baked Potato Chips, cheese and onion

1 mini pitta dipped in 2 tbsp light fromage frais mixed with 1 level tbsp grated Parmesan cheese

1 × 25g bag Twiglets

If you want something **SPICY**, forget the take-away curry or chilli ...

For **25 calories** or less	For **50 calories** or less	For **100 calories** or less
Spring onions dipped into WeightWatchers Mayonnaise Dressing laced with chilli powder	1 dark rye Ryvita spread with any brand hot salsa dip	1 mini pitta sliced with Old El Paso hot salsa
	1 Slice a Rice topped with plenty of ready hot and spicy salsa	1 pack WeightWatchers Cheese Dippers
	1 Sharwood's Ready to Eat large spiced poppadom with 1 tbsp ready salsa	25g pretzels

If you want something **STARCHY**, leave the gâteau or the doughnut and go for ...

For **25 calories** or less	For **50 calories** or less	For **100 calories** or less
1 Amaretti biscuit	1 Jaffa cake	1 mini white pitta with 1 tsp low-sugar jam
1 tsp cooked rice	1 slice wholemeal bread from a small sliced loaf with a little low fat spread	Average slice bread from large sliced loaf with low-fat spread and low-sugar jam
		Round crumpet with low-fat spread
		Medium slice malt loaf with low-fat spread
		1 large banana

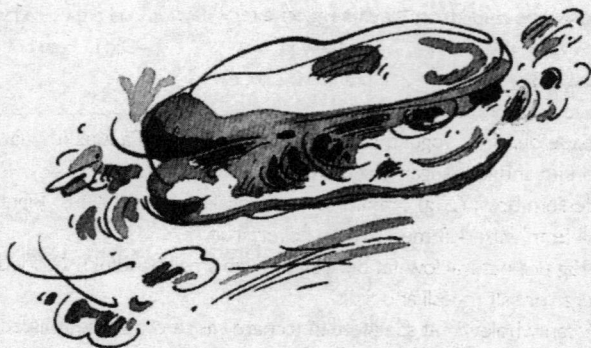

WEEK ONE

Notes

- For instructions, allowances and 'unlimiteds', see pages 28–9.
- Don't forget to add unlimited vegetable and salad items to your meals whenever you can.
- Don't forget to fill up on your daily Snack Swaps and your daily Fruit Snack.
- Don't forget your Week's Treats too!
- When **BREAD** is mentioned in the diet, unless otherwise stated it is a slice from a medium-cut large sliced loaf.
- If **FRUIT** is mentioned within a meal but not specified, choose any fresh, frozen or canned in juice fruit, which can be either 1 whole medium fruit, 2 small fruits, 1 small banana, a large bowlful of berries, a small bowlful of mixed fruit salad or a ringpull can of Fruitini. Do not use dried fruit unless specified and avoid fruit canned in syrup.
- You will be pleased to see that weighing and measuring have been avoided when possible through the use of single-portion items, and spoons.

Choose one meal from each section every day.

BREAKFASTS

- Shape diet fruit yogurt; 1 apple; 1 slice bread with a little low-fat spread and low-sugar jam, marmalade or Marmite.
- Medium bowl (25g) branflakes or cornflakes, Special K, Just Right or All-Bran with skimmed milk to cover; fruit.
- 125g pot natural low-fat bio yogurt with small handful no added sugar or salt muesli and fruit.
- ½ can wholewheat spaghetti in tomato sauce on 1 slice toasted bread, with a little low-fat spread.
- 1 Shape Greek Style lemon yoghurt; 1 large banana.

LUNCHES PACKED

- 2 slices bread with a little low-fat spread filled with 1 individual portion Bel Paese cream cheese or 2 slices extra-lean ham, 2 teaspoons sweet pickle, lettuce; 1 individual pot any low fat fruit fromage frais; 1 portion fruit.
- 1 white pitta filled with 1 × 100g can tuna in brine, drained, mixed with 1 tablespoon WeightWatchers Mayonnaise Dressing and chopped crisp raw vegetables/salad of choice; 1 Shape fruit yogurt.

LUNCHES HOME

- ½ 400g can baked beans in tomato sauce on 1 slice toast, with a little low-fat spread, topped with 1 level tablespoon grated half-fat cheese; 1 large banana.
- 1 Findus French Bread Pizza, ham and pineapple or cheese and tomato flavour; 1 individual pot any low fat fruit fromage frais; fruit.
- Ten-calorie soup (optional); cooked chicken breast portion with unlimited salad items of choice; small wholemeal roll and low-fat spread.

LUNCHES TAKEOUT

- Any supermarket calorie-counted sandwich 300 calories or less; fruit.
- McDonald's hamburger (regular, no cheese); McDonald's pure orange juice.

EVENING MEALS MAKE-AHEAD MEALS

- Tarragon Pork (see recipe page 45).
- Chicken and Mushroom Pancakes (see recipe page 44).

EVENING MEALS REAL MEALS IN MOMENTS

- If you have any leftover cooked potatoes plus eggs – Spanish Omelette (see recipe page 49).
- 1 average turkey fillet, grilled or fried using a little Fry Light spray in a non-stick pan; large portion frozen mixed vegetables; 4 tablespoons mashed potato (instant if liked, or mashed using skimmed milk); 1 dessertspoon relish of choice.
- 50g (dry weight) couscous, reconstituted according to pack instructions and topped with 1 whole 340–400g can ratatouille plus 2 tablespoons grated Parmesan cheese.

EVENING MEALS READY MEALS

(Do have plenty of your unlimited vegetable/salad with any selection from here.)
- Any ready to eat single-portion chicken curry with rice OR Vegetable lasagne containing 400 calories or less.
- St Michael Cannelloni (285g).
- Birds Eye Roast Beef or Turkey Platter.

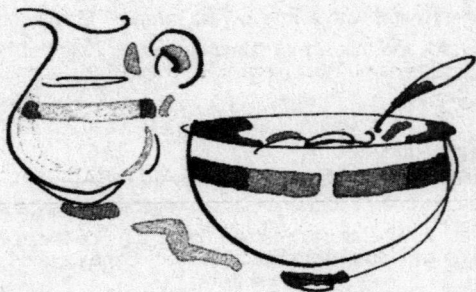

WEEK **TWO**

Notes

As Week 1 plus:
* Don't forget to read through your meal options and plan ahead for the week. It'll save you time and hunger!

BREAKFASTS

* 1 Müller Fruit Corner yoghurt plus one apple.
* 2 slices bread or toast with low-fat spread and low-sugar jam or marmalade or Marmite.
* 2 Weetabix with skimmed milk to cover; 1 small glass grapefruit juice.
* 125ml low-fat natural bio yogurt; 1 small banana; 1 teaspoon honey.

LUNCHES PACKED

* 2 slices bread spread with WeightWatchers Mayonnaise Dressing and filled with unlimited salad plus 2 slices lean turkey from vacuum pack, 2 tsp cranberry sauce (optional); 1 Jordan's Fruesli Bar.
* 3 dark rye Ryvitas with a little low-fat spread; 1 Camembert triangle (pick and mix size); 1 tomato; 1 apple; 200g pot Müller Light yogurt.

LUNCHES HOME

* 1 whole carton New Covent Garden vegetable soup (any variety e.g. Tomato and Lentil or Leek and Potato); 1 slice bread with low-fat spread.
* Large egg poached on 1 slice toast with low-fat spread; 2 satsumas; Quaker Harvest Chewy bar.

LUNCHES TAKEOUT

- Take-away baked potato with baked bean filling; fruit.
- Small baguette or soft wholemeal bap filled with chicken and salad (no mayonnaise).
- Boots Shapers Wrap, any variety; kiwi or satsuma or plum.

EVENING MEALS MAKE-AHEAD MEALS

- Balti Curry (see recipe page 46).
- Penne Primavera (see recipe page 48).

EVENING MEALS REAL MEALS IN MOMENTS

- Individual portion frozen cod fillet in breadcrumbs, grilled; 100g pack McCain Micro Chips, heated in microwave; grilled tomato; 3 tablespoons frozen petit pois or peas, boiled or microwaved.
- If you have a selection of sweet peppers – Stir-fried Peppers and Egg (see recipe page 50).
- Pitta pizza – Heat grill; spread 1 tablespoon sundried tomato paste *or* some ready-made Italian Tomato Sauce over one side of a pitta bread; top with sliced tomato and finely chopped onion and seasoning, and top that with 2 level tablespoons grated half-fat mozzarella (available in resealable freezable packs). Grill until bubbling and serve with salad.

EVENING MEALS READY MEALS

- Indian take-away vegetable curry with plain boiled rice.
- Chilled or frozen individual size Fisherman's Pie (about 300g); salad; 2 tablespoons peas.
- WeightWatchers Beef Lasagne; salad.

WEEK **THREE**

Notes

As Week 1 plus:

- If you like you can choose a meal option from another week – as long as you swap breakfast for breakfast, lunch for lunch, and so on.
- Don't forget to take plenty of exercise.

BREAKFASTS

- Large boiled egg; 1 slice bread or toast with a little low-fat spread; small glass grapefruit juice.
- 1 individual box Kelloggs' cereal from pick and mix selection with skimmed milk to cover; fruit.
- 1 Nutri-Grain morning bar; 1 Shape fruit yogurt or 1 portion fruit.

LUNCHES PACKED

- 2 slices bread with a little low-fat spread filled with 2 slices lean chicken from vacuum pack and salad plus 1 dessertspoon WeightWatchers Mayonnaise Dressing; 1 large banana.
- 1 can of John West Tuna Light Meal; 1 individual pot any low fat fruit fromage frais; 1 portion fruit.

LUNCHES AT HOME

- 275g baked potato filled with 100g pot ready-made tzatziki; salad or fruit.
- 1/2 medium ripe avocado filled with oil-free French dressing or a dash of balsamic vinegar; salad; 1 small wholemeal roll with a little low-fat spread; 1 Shape fruit yogurt.

LUNCHES TAKEOUT

- 1 portion pasta salad with mushrooms and tomato sauce.
- 1 reduced-calorie sandwich 300 calories or less; 1 portion fruit.

EVENING MEALS MAKE-AHEAD MEALS

- Salmon with Pesto and Spaghetti (see recipe page 43).
- Sweet and Sour Pork and Noodles (see recipe page 47).

EVENING MEALS REAL MEALS IN MOMENTS

- From the store-cupboard – Pasta with Sardines and Sultanas (see recipe page 42).
- Chicken tacos – slice 1 chicken breast fillet and microwave or stir-fry in Old El Paso mild or hot taco sauce until cooked through; use to fill 2 taco shells with chopped crisp lettuce, tomato, onion. Top with 1 tablespoon ready-made guacamole (avocado purée/dip)* or with 1 tablespoon Greek yogurt or half-fat crème fraîche.

EVENING MEALS READY MEALS

- Any ready to eat single-portion vegetable curry with rice; 1 dessertspoon sweet mango chutney; fruit OR. Chicken and vegetable stir-fry containing 400 calories or less; 1 dessertspoon mango chutney; salad.
- Vegetable and pasta bake; 1 tablespoon grated half-fat Cheddar over top; fruit or Shape fruit yogurt.
- ½ average 2-portion cheese and tomato pizza.

* FROM DELI COUNTER OR IN JARS FROM MOST SUPERMARKETS.

20 QUICK AND EASY RECIPES

PASTA WITH SARDINES AND SULTANAS

(Real Meals in Moments, Week 3)
10 minutes to prepare and cook

Serves 1
470 calories and 21g fat per portion

40g (dry weight) spaghettini or other thin pasta
1 dessertspoon olive oil
2 spring onions, sliced into thin rounds
4 canned sardines, well drained and dried with
kitchen paper
1 level tablespoon sultanas
1 level dessertspoon pine nuts
A dash of lemon juice
1 tablespoon fresh parsley or 1 teaspoon freeze-dried
A little salt and black pepper

Boil some water in a kettle and fill a saucepan, bring back to boil; add the pasta and a dash of salt. Boil, uncovered, for 10 minutes or as pack instructs.

Meanwhile, heat the oil in a small non-stick frying pan and stir in the onions. Chop each sardine into four and when the onions are slightly soft, add them to the pan with the sultanas and pine nuts. Stir very gently for a minute, adding the lemon juice, parsley and seasoning half way through. When the pasta is ready, drain and serve with the sardine sauce lightly combined.

SALMON WITH CHILLI AND SPAGHETTI

(Make-Ahead Meal, Week 3)
25 minutes to prepare and cook; will freeze

Serves 2
402 calories and 16.5g fat per portion

175g salmon fillet
Fry Light spray
1 large red pepper
250ml and ready-made tomato and chilli sauce
80g (dry weight) tagliatelle or spaghetti
Basil leaves, to garnish (optional)

Heat a medium non-stick frying pan (which has a lid) sprayed well with Fry Light. Chop the salmon into bite-sized cubes and add to the pan, stirring gently until lightly golden. Remove with a slotted spoon and set aside. Deseed and thinly slice the pepper and stir for 2 minutes in the pan with more Fry Light added. Add the sauce to the pan, turn the heat down and simmer, covered, for 20 minutes or until the peppers are fairly tender. Add the salmon for the last 2 minutes of cooking.

Meanwhile, cook the tagliatelle in boiling salted water and drain.

Arrange the pasta in two freezerproof, microwaveproof lidded single-serving dishes and top with the sauce. To serve, reheat in the microwave until piping hot and garnish with fresh basil if liked.

CHICKEN AND MUSHROOM PANCAKES

(Make-Ahead Meals, Week 1)
10 minutes to prepare and cook; will freeze

Serves 2
445 calories and 14g fat per portion

200g stir-fry lean chicken pieces
Fry Light spray
200g small firm tasty mushrooms
1 × 50g pack Knorr Parsley Sauce mix
100g frozen sweetcorn or petit pois, defrosted (see note)
Salt and pepper
4 medium ready-to-eat pancakes (see note)
Fresh parsley (optional)

Heat a non-stick frying pan sprayed with Fry Light and add the chicken in one layer. Leave until the underneath is golden, then turn the pieces over and repeat (if you try to stir them about until they are sealed, they will stick!).

Remove the pan from the heat. Cut the mushrooms into thin slices and make up the parsley sauce according to pack instructions. Add the sauce, mushrooms, sweetcorn and seasoning to the pan, stir well and bring to a simmer for 2–3 minutes. Spoon a quarter of the sauce into the middle of each pancake and roll up or fold into quarters.

Carefully place into one or two freezerproof, ovenproof/microwave-proof dish/es of suitable size, sprinkle with parsley if using and chill or freeze. Reheat in the microwave or oven until filling is bubbling.

NOTE *Sweetcorn or peas can be defrosted in moments either by placing in a sieve and running water over them, or in the microwave. Ready-made thin pancakes (crêpes) can be bought in packs from most supermarkets; find them near the breads. Any surplus pancakes can be frozen.*

TARRAGON PORK

(Make-Ahead Meals, Week 1)
15 minutes to prepare and cook; will freeze

Serves 2
382 calories and 14g fat per portion

75g pasta shapes of choice
1 dessertspoon corn oil
8 shallots, halved
225g pork tenderloin
25ml dry white wine
25ml full-fat crème fraîche
1 tablespoon fresh chopped tarragon
(or 1 dessertspoon freeze-dried)
Salt and pepper

Boil a kettle of water and fill a saucepan, add the pasta with a little salt and cook until tender – about 12 minutes. Drain.

Meanwhile, heat the oil in a non-stick frying pan and add the shallots to fry, stirring from time to time, over a medium heat. Slice the pork tenderloin into 1cm thick slices and when the shallots are beginning to brown, after about 5 minutes, add the pork to the pan. Cook to brown each side, then add the wine, lower the heat and simmer for 2–3 minutes. Add the crème fraîche, tarragon and seasoning, stir well and serve with the pasta.

BALTI CURRY

(Make-Ahead Meals, Week 2)
25 minutes to prepare and cook; will freeze

Serves 2
418 calories and 15g fat per portion

60g (dry weight) basmati rice
175g extra-lean minced beef
1 medium onion
1 small (about 150g) aubergine
2 whole tomatoes (canned, drained or fresh, skinned)
100g baby spinach or spring greens or French beans
200ml Chicken Tonight or Homepride Balti Sauce
2 tablespoons low-fat natural yogurt

Put the rice on to simmer in a little lightly salted water according to pack instructions.

Meanwhile, put the meat in a non-stick frying pan and slowly heat, stirring from time to time, gradually increasing heat so that the fat runs out (which it will even with lean meat) and the meat begins to brown.

Meanwhile, finely slice and chop the onion. When the meat is browned, remove it from the pan with a slotted spoon and reserve. In the remaining fat, sauté the onion, stirring from time to time, until transparent and turning golden. While the onion is cooking, chop the aubergine into 1cm rounds and then each into a quarter, and quarter the tomatoes. Add both to the pan and stir-fry with the onions for a few minutes. Add the spinach to the pan and stir. (If using spring greens, shred them finely.) Return the meat to the pan with the sauce, stir, bring to a simmer and cook, stirring frequently, for a few minutes.

Spoon the cooked rice into two individual, freezerproof, ovenproof/microwaveproof lidded containers and spoon the curry on top. Freeze or chill and reheat thoroughly, before serving drizzled with the yogurt.

NOTE *Fresh coriander leaves sprinkled on top are very good. You can serve the Balti curry with mini pitta breads instead of the rice if you like, in which case you can add a dessertspoon of mango chutney per serving, if you want.*

SWEET AND SOUR PORK AND NOODLES

(Make-Ahead Meals, Week 3)
20 minutes to prepare and cook; will freeze

Serves 2
413 calories and 9g fat per portion

75g (dry weight) fine egg thread noodles
1 dessertspoon groundnut oil
1 medium onion or 6 spring onions, halved lengthways
200g lean pork fillet
1 medium carrot
1 small yellow pepper
50g Chinese leaves or Cos lettuce
50g beansprouts
160g jar Sharwood's Sweet and Sour Sauce

Pour boiling water over the noodles in a pan and leave to soften according to pack instructions; drain.

Meanwhile, heat the oil in non-stick frying pan and stir-fry the onion until turning golden. Cut the pork into thin strips and add it to the pan, stirring until brown. Slice the carrot and yellow pepper into thin strips and add to the pan, stirring again for a few minutes, adding a little water or chicken stock if the pan gets too dry. Add the Chinese leaves, beansprouts and sauce and stir for 2 minutes. Arrange the noodles in two individual, lidded, freezerproof, ovenproof/microwaveproof dishes and spoon the pork sauce on top. Freeze or chill. Reheat thoroughly.

NOTE *If you don't want to use beansprouts, increase the amount of Chinese leaves or Cos instead.*

PENNE PRIMAVERA

(Make-Ahead Meals, Week 2)
20 minutes to prepare and cook; will freeze

Serves 2
400 calories and 10g fat per portion

150g (dry weight) penne pasta tricolor
1 medium courgette
50g sugarsnap peas or baby sweetcorn
1 dessertspoon olive oil
2 medium leeks
100g firm mushrooms
1 teaspoon garlic purée
75ml passata
Salt and black pepper
2 level tablespoons half-fat crème fraîche
2 tablespoons grated Parmesan cheese

Cook the pasta in boiling, lightly salted water until cooked; drain.
Meanwhile, thinly slice the courgette and parboil the courgette slices and sugarsnaps or sweetcorn for 2 minutes, drain; pat dry on kitchen paper. Heat the oil in a non-stick frying pan. While it is heating, slice the leeks thinly, then add to the pan and stir until beginning to soften. Thinly slice the mushrooms. Add the courgette, peas, mushrooms and garlic purée and stir for 2–3 minutes. Add the passata and seasoning and simmer for a further 2–3 minutes. Stir in the crème fraîche and then, when the pasta is cooked, mix the sauce with the pasta and top with the cheese. Spoon into two lidded individual, freezerproof ovenproof/microwaveproof containers and freeze or chill. Reheat thoroughly before serving.

SPANISH OMELETTE

(Real Meals in Moments, Week 1)
10 minutes to prepare and cook

Serves 1
408 calories and 18g fat per portion

2 large eggs
Salt and pepper
1 teaspoon corn or olive oil
100g leftover cooked potato
3 spring onions
1 slice bread, toasted, with a little low-fat spread

In a bowl, beat the eggs with a little cold water and salt and pepper. Heat the oil in a small non-stick frying pan.

Meanwhile, slice the potato thinly and chop the spring onions. When the pan is hot, add the eggs to the pan and arrange the potato slices and onions around the pan evenly. Cook over a low to medium heat until the underside of the egg is golden. Flash the pan under the grill to brown the top or place an inverted plate over the top of the pan and turn the omelette over to cook the other side. Serve when both sides are set and golden, with the toast and plenty of salad.

STIR-FRIED PEPPERS AND EGG

(Real Meals in Moments, Week 2)
15 minutes to prepare and cook

Serves 1
395 calories and 19g fat per portion

1 tablespoon olive oil
200g mixed peppers
1 small onion
1 fresh tomato
1 pinch ground chilli
Salt and black pepper
1 large egg
1 mini pitta

Heat the olive oil in a medium non-stick frying pan.

Meanwhile, deseed the peppers and very thinly slice both them and the onion. Add to the pan and stir-fry for 7–8 minutes until soft and tinged golden. Chop the tomato (deseeded if you like) and add it to the pan with the chilli and seasoning. Poach the egg and heat the pitta. Serve the cooked pepper mixture topped with the poached egg and with the pitta.

Alternatively, you could transfer the pepper mixture into a microwaveproof or ovenproof dish, break the egg on top and cook in the oven for 10 minutes or so, or in the microwave for 90 seconds or so, until the egg white is cooked but the yolk still soft. This will add to the length of cooking time.

the sweet-tooth plan

Y ou want to lose weight. But you have a sweet tooth. You can't live without chocolate, or your daily biscuit fix or your regular cream cake treat – and you don't want to try.

So you don't bother trying to lose weight. It's impossible.

Well, I think you are wrong. You can slim down and still have a daily fix of sweet food; you can even have chocolate bars and those cream cakes on a regular basis.

The trick is to keep your body and your mind happy on amounts of these items which will still have you losing weight. The trick is also to get rid of the guilt that so often accompanies a sweet tooth. This chapter is all about showing you how to do these things.

Why do we have a sweet tooth?

It is often said that a sweet tooth is inborn, and that could be the case. Breast milk is sweet, which could be one reason why most children enjoy sweets and sweet foods, and why many never grow out of this.

Breast milk is also fatty. One of our main sweet-tooth addictions is for another sweet and fatty item – chocolate. And this could explain at least partly why chocolate is our number one food addiction. Chocolate is also rich in caffeine, a stimulant, phenylethylamine, a hormone linked to arousal, and theobromine, another stimulant. No wonder that chocolate has been estimated as being the downfall of around 60 per cent of all slimming diets!

Other reasons that so many of us love sweet foods are that they are easy to eat and they are instant gratification. And one scientific reason is that most sweet foods create an almost immediate increase in blood sugar levels – a sugar craving can be caused by low blood sugar and the physical feeling that you 'need something sweet'.

Are sweet foods really that bad?

The World Health Organisation recently confirmed that sugar and sweet foods **ARE HEALTHY** in moderation – up to 10 per cent of our daily calories can come from sugars. On a slimming diet such as in this chapter that means you could have 130 calories' worth, or nearly 35 grams of sugar a day. But as we have seen, sweet foods are almost always (with the exception of some confectionery and ice lollies) high or quite high in fat. It is the fat content of these items that, in the minds of most nutritionists, gives most cause for concern, as the fat in sweet foods is often saturated (the kind linked with heart disease) and a high-fat diet is also linked with weight gain and many other problems.

The World Health Organisation sets a reasonable target for daily fat intake of 30 per cent of total calories. On the slimming diet in this chapter that would represent 390 calories' worth of fat, or 43g of fat. A target of 10 per cent of total calories maximum in the form of saturated fat is reasonable, so on this diet, you can have 130 calories' worth of saturated fat a day, or 14.5g.

So how can I eat sweet/fatty foods on your diet?

What I have done is give you a weekly 'sweet treats' guideline of 1,400 calories (or an average of 200 calories a day) for sweet/fatty foods. As below, you will see you can have up to four sweet snacks a day on such a plan, so it is quite a generous allowance.

I have done this by making absolutely sure that the rest of your day's diet – a breakfast, lunch, evening meal, milk allowance and snack – is low in fat and sugar. Breakfasts contain 4g of fat or less; lunches 8g of fat or less; evening meals 12g of fat or less; your milk is virtually fat-free and your snack 2g of fat or less. This all adds up to a maximum of 26g fat a day, leaving you with 17g fat a day to 'spend' on sweet treats. I have also pared down the saturated fat in the daily meals to the minimum so that much of the 17g fat for your treat can be in the form of saturated fat.

Your daily sugar maximum allowance of 35g is more than enough to cover any sweet treat you're likely to eat. So that is how it is done!

Eating 'treat' foods is fine – as long as you keep your overall diet in balance and keep in mind my four easy steps to being boss of your own sweet tooth.

Four easy steps to Sweet-tooth success

Keep your body happy

To help prevent low blood sugar you need to feed your body frequently, which is why my plan offers three meals and one healthy snack a day as well as your sweet treats. Never go more than four hours without a meal or snack while you slim. Your ideal eating pattern on this diet may be breakfast between 8 and 9am; lunch between 12 and 1pm, healthy snack about 4–4.30pm, and evening meal about 7–8pm (although if you have particular 'danger times' – see below – you may want to adjust these). In between meals you can snack on any of the 'unlimited' items (see page 56) and you also have your daily sweet treats **BUT** it is important **NOT** to eat high-sugar sweet treats when you feel very hungry and haven't eaten for a while. If you do, you may well find you eat much more than you'd planned. Try to eat your sweet treats either with a meal or snack, or soon after a meal or snack. That way you will find it much easier to eat no more than you had planned and you won't overstep your weekly allowance.

The meals and snacks within the Sweet-tooth Plan also have one other advantage – they are high in foods which take a long time to be absorbed into the bloodstream and which will keep you feeling full for longer, and keep your blood sugar levels on a more even keel.

It is important to eat everything you are allowed on the plan.

Some of you will have been eating much more sweet/fatty foods than you are allowed on this plan. If you eat as explained above, spacing meals out well, you shouldn't find this a problem, but if you get sweet cravings **DON'T** snack on high-calorie chocolate bars (outside your weekly allowance) but have an extra Healthy Snack, an apple, an orange, or a little dried fruit.

As explained above, when you eat high-sugar foods in between meals, your blood sugar levels tend to fluctuate, possibly causing you to crave the very foods you should be avoiding.

Keep your mind happy

You need to get your head right if you are going to follow this plan happily. That means admitting that you aren't going to die if you get less than your usual amount of sweets or chocolates. It means admitting that you need to pay more attention to what you are putting in your mouth. And it means becoming a bit of a detective in spotting likely times and situations when you would normally have something sweet and fattening without even thinking about it – and lining up an alternative strategy.

I would like you to keep a diary for a week of what you eat, and every time you eat something sweet, write down why. A pattern will emerge of your danger times – both hungry times of day and times when you're eating for reasons other than hunger (of which there will be many).

Adjust your daily mealtimes to ensure that your hungriest times of day are catered for, and think up at least 10 strategies or alternatives to pigging out on sweet foods when you need comfort, when you're bored, or whatever your own danger moments are. These should be simple, immediate and non-expensive things like taking a bath, phoning a friend, going for a walk, watching a favourite video and so on.

Don't forget that eating to slim begins in the shop. What you don't buy you can't eat – so when possible plan all your meals and your sweet treats for the week, buying only what you need. If you have a family and they eat a lot of sweet food too, they could do worse than cut down with you, so if they moan because the cake tin isn't laden, for instance, tell them they will have to buy and eat their sweet foods outside the home in future!

Get rid of the guilt

The art of eating is to enjoy every last mouthful. You can't do that if you're riddled with guilt about it. So don't forget that on this plan your sweet foods are allowed, are included within your diet, are there to be savoured with not a shred of guilt at all.

Every day, plan when you are going to have your sweet treats, look forward to this and tell yourself you deserve it. This is the good way to think. If you feel guilty, there's no point.

This is especially important for anyone who has been on the binge/starve pattern. You start a diet, giving up all your favourite foods, but after a few days (or whatever) you get a massive urge to binge, do so, then feel guilty and either give up all thoughts of slimming (if you're very overweight, bad), or feel guilty and try to starve yourself (worse).

If for now you think of sweet foods as something to be enjoyed, maybe before long you will be able to think of chocolate, or whatever your treat is, as a regular part of your diet. A food that is no more important or less important than potatoes or meat or bread or milk. It's just part of your varied healthy eating plan. In other words, you like it, it's there, but it's not worth losing sleep over.

When you can get to that stage, you are in control of your sweet tooth; it isn't controlling you.

Get a life

Sweet foods aren't the be-all and end-all of life.

I have written this plan because I would rather you lose weight with sweet foods than stay fat with sweet foods. And, at the moment, you feel there is no option.

But in the long term, sweets and cakes and chocolates aren't what you need for a happy life. Your body doesn't actually need them at all. It needs a balanced healthy diet, which may include a caramel bar or a cream doughnut – but it may not.

A strange thing may happen along the way when you follow this plan. You may come to agree with me, and realise that you can go for a day or two, or more, without a sweet fix. Partly this will be because you're eating an overall more healthy, regular, varied and balanced diet. And partly this will be because your food diary and your own thoughts are making you realise that sweet treats have been taking the place of other, better things in life – like exercise, activity, fun, fashion, achievement, friends, new plans or even regular time to yourself.

Or they have been taking the place of action and therapy to sort out life's problems, such as relationship difficulties, work stress or lack of confidence. When people have problems in life, they don't turn to cabbage or skimmed milk, they turn to sweet foods. In other words, the last step to controlling your sweet food need is to begin to change not just your diet, but your life. Start making some plans now.

What to do

Read the following pages before beginning the plan.

Unlimiteds

Every day on the diet you can have the following items in addition to what is listed within the meals:

- **Drinks** Water, mineral water, diet fizzy drinks, low-calorie squashes, tea or coffee (black or with milk from allowance and with artificial sweetener – or sugar as part of daily treat, see below), herb teas, unsweetened fruit teas.
- **Foods** Salad vegetables, leafy green vegetables.
- **Condiments** Fresh or dried herbs and spices, lemon juice, lime juice, Worcestershire sauce, light soy sauce, tomato purée, passata, vinegar, oil-free dressings.

Milk Allowance

Every day you have an allowance of 250ml skimmed milk or 200ml semi-skimmed milk for use in tea or coffee or as a drink on its own. If not required, have one 125ml pot natural low-fat yogurt instead for the calcium content. Milk for breakfast cereals is on top of this allowance.

Meals and Snacks

Every day during the three weeks, pick one Breakfast, one Lunch, one Evening Meal and one Healthy Snack from the options given each week.

Sweet Treats

Every week you have an allowance of 1,400 calories 'spare' so that you can choose whatever sweet treats you like to that value. This should preferably be used as 200 calories a day, certainly for the first two weeks of the plan. On pages 59–60 are my Top 40 selections for you to choose from; these vary in calories from 50 through to 200 so you can decide how you want to use your allowance – e.g. 4 × 50 calorie treats a day; 2 × 50 plus 1 × 100 calorie treats a day; 2 × 100 calorie treats a day; 1 × 50 and 1 × 150 calorie treats a day, or 1 × 200 calorie treat a day. It is up to you.

You could instead choose from the 'under 150' or 'under 200' calorie sweet recipes on pages 67–72 or you could turn to pages 76–8 for more branded sweet foods information. If you fancy something savoury, or a glass of wine or beer, or a knob of butter, or whatever, instead – feel free to have it instead of something sweet, as long as you are sure of the exact calorie count. As long as your extras add up to no more than 200 a day, you will still lose weight.

Many branded desserts and yogurts, and other foods, give calorie information on their packs so you aren't just limited to what you can find in this book.

In the later weeks of the diet plan, you can be more flexible with your 1,400 calories a week without the need to divide this up into 200 calories a day. For instance, you might decide to have 4 × 300 calorie treats on four days plus 2 × 100 calorie treats on two days, or whatever. This will mean you can include any of the higher-calorie recipe dishes on pages 73–5, and more of the items listed on pages 76–8. But using the whole 1,400 calories up in one day isn't advisable – try to spread it out.

Eat sweet treats with, or soon after, a meal. Remember – don't feel guilty; this allowance forms a legitimate part of your overall healthy slimming plan.

Fill out the diary. Every week there is space for you to fill in your sweet treats so that there is no chance of you forgetting what you've had. Do fill it in – it will help.

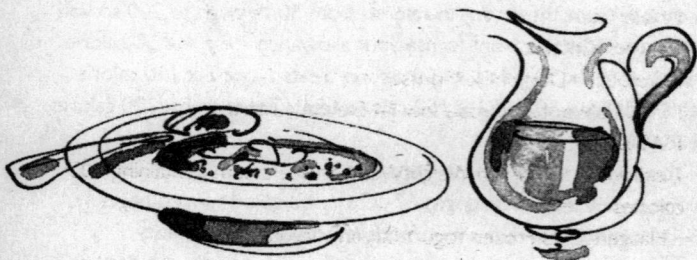

40 Sweet Snacks You Can Enjoy Without Guilt

Use these snacks as part of your Sweet-tooth Plan, the instructions for which appear on the previous page.

50 calories or less

- 1 dark rye Ryvita spread generously with chocolate spread, any variety.
- 1 WeightWatchers Real Chocolate Chip Cookie.
- 1 sachet instant low-fat hot chocolate drink, any variety, made up.
- Up to 1 whole sachet sugar-free jelly (up to a pint).
- 1 Yoplait Frubes 40g tube.
- 3 rounded teaspoonfuls sugar (for use in tea or coffee).

100 calories or less

- 1 × 2-pack WeightWatchers cookies, any variety.
- 1 Go Ahead Caramel Crisp bar.
- 1 Quaker Harvest Chewy Bar, any variety
- 1 round crumpet generously spread with low-sugar jam.
- 1 Halo bar.
- 2 fingers KitKat.
- 1 Cadbury's Dairy Milk Mousse.
- 1 individual pot Ambrosia low-fat Devon custard.
- 1 Walls Twister.
- 1 individual 100ml tub WeightWatchers ice cream containing 100 calories or less
- 1 Häagen-Dazs Frozen Yogurt bar, any flavour

150 calories or less

- I Hob Nob individual bar.
- I Shepherdboy Apple Fruit and Nut bar.
- I Cadbury's Caramel cake bar.
- I Mr Kipling Almond Slice.
- I Lyons Cup Cake, any variety.
- I Lyons Jam Tart.
- I individual pot Ambrosia Creamed Rice or custard (full fat).
- Any individual chilled or frozen dessert containing 150 calories or less (e.g. Cadbury's Original Mousse, any Boots Shapers Dessert)

200 calories or less

- I Mars Tracker Choc Chip.
- I Rowntree's Chunky Aero bar.
- I Cadbury's Crunchie bar.
- I Cadbury's Creme Egg.
- I Cadbury's Wispa bar.
- I Mr Kipling Strawberry Sundae or Cherry Bakewell.
- I Cadbury's Caramel ice cream.
- I Wall's Strawberry Cornetto.

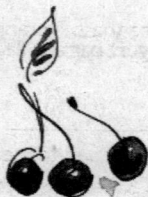

WEEK **ONE**

Notes

- Don't forget your 'Unlimiteds' and Sweet Treats (see pages 56–8).
- Unless otherwise stated, bread is 1 slice of brown, white or wholemeal bread from a large, medium-cut sliced loaf and it is very lightly spread with low-fat spread.
- Try to vary your meal choices as much as possible.

BREAKFASTS

- 25g All-Bran with 125ml skimmed milk and 1 medium banana.
- 1 slice bread or toast with low-sugar jam or marmalade; 1 Shape diet fruit yogurt; 1 plum, nectarine or satsuma.
- 25g cornflakes with 125ml skimmed milk and 40g ready-to-eat dried apricots (5 apricot pieces), chopped in.

LUNCHES

- Sandwich of 2 slices bread filled with 40g low-fat soft cheese and salad; 1 apple.
- 1 whole carton any New Covent Garden or other chilled fresh soup containing 250 calories or less; 1 slice bread; 1 kiwifruit or satsuma.
- 1 small wholemeal roll with a very little low-fat spread; 1 medium cooked chicken breast portion, skin removed; fresh salad selection with oil-free French dressing or balsamic vinegar; medium slice melon or 1 plum.
- 200g baked beans on 1 slice toast; 1 orange or 2 satsumas.

EVENING MEALS

- 50g (dry weight) pasta cooked and topped with 4 tablespoons ready-made Italian Tomato Sauce plus 1 tablespoon grated Parmesan cheese; large side salad; small apple.

- 200g white fish steak or fillet, grilled, microwaved or baked; 150g new or boiled potatoes; 3 tablespoons peas; 1 level dessertspoon tomato sauce or WeightWatchers Mayonnaise Dressing; 1 medium banana.
- 1 × 150g turkey fillet, sliced and stir-fried with a selection of thinly sliced fresh vegetables in 1 dessertspoon oil with light soy sauce and 1 level dessertspoon Sharwood's Hoi Sin Sauce and chicken stock as necessary; 3 tablespoons cooked rice.
- 1 portion Tarragon Pork (see recipe page 45).
- Any individual ready-to-eat chicken meal containing 400 calories or less; 1 apple.

HEALTHY SNACKS

- 1 large banana.
- 5 ready-to-eat stoned prunes; 1 apple.
- 15g shelled sunflower seeds.
- 125g pot Danone Bio Yogurt Lite, any flavour.

SWEET TREATS RECORD

	Had	Calories	Running Total
Monday			
Tuesday			
Wednesday			
Thursday			
Friday			
Saturday			
Sunday			
Week Total			1,400 calories

WEEK **TWO**

Notes

- Try to space your meals out evenly.
- Remember to eat Sweet Treats with or shortly after a meal or snack.

BREAKFASTS

- 1 large banana; 1 × 200g pot Müller Light banana or vanilla yogurt.
- 1 Nutri-Grain morning bar, blueberry or strawberry; 1 Shape Fruit Juice Mousse.
- 1 slice toast, with Marmite; 25g All-Bran with milk from allowance; 1 plum, satsuma or kiwi fruit.

LUNCHES

- Sandwich of 2 slices bread filled with 1 medium hard-boiled egg, 1 teaspoon WeightWatchers Mayonnaise Dressing and salad; 1 apple.
- 1 whole carton any New Covent Garden or other chilled fresh soup containing 200 calories or less; 1 mini pitta; kiwi fruit.
- Any individual vegetable curry or vegetable stir-fry ready to eat meal containing 300 calories or less; salad.
- 1 pot Phileas Fogg BBQ Dip with selection of vegetable crudités plus 2 crisprolls (e.g. Sunblest);
  1 Shape raspberry and white chocolate yoghurt.

EVENING MEALS

- 1 × 225g baked potato; 1 medium chicken breast portion, baked in foil with lemon juice, herbs and seasoning; 3 tablespoons sweetcorn, 1 portion 'unlimited' leafy greens.
- Salmon with Chilli and Spaghetti (see recipe page 43).
- Tarragon Pork (see recipe page 45).

- Any individual ready-to-eat pasta meal containing 400 calories or less; large mixed salad.
- Macaroni cheese made (for one portion) with 50g macaroni, cooked and mixed with quarter pack Napolina Creamy Bake Lasagne Sauce plus 75g cooked broccoli florets and garnished with 1 sliced tomato and 25g grated half-fat mozzarella cheese. (If serving more, simply multiply the ingredients accordingly.)

HEALTHY SNACKS

- 1 slice of bread with pure fruit spread.
- 1 Shape Fruit Juice Mousse, plum and blackcurrant flavour.
- 1 mini pitta filled with salad items and oil-free French dressing or balsamic vinegar.

SWEET TREATS RECORD

	Had	Calories	Running Total
Monday			
Tuesday			
Wednesday			
Thursday			
Friday			
Saturday			
Sunday			
Week Total			1,400 calories

WEEK **THREE**

NOTES

- Don't forget to include plenty of 'unlimited' vegetables with your evening meals and salad stuff with your lunches.
- You can choose meals from other weeks in the programme to vary your diet more, as long as you pick one Breakfast, one Lunch, one Evening Meal and one Healthy Snack a day.

BREAKFASTS

- 2–3 large tomatoes, quartered and grilled or dry-fried in a non-stick pan with Fry Light spray, served on 1 $\frac{1}{2}$ slices toast; with 1 level tablespoon grated Parmesan cheese sprinkled over.
- 40g no added sugar or salt muesli with 100ml skimmed milk and $\frac{1}{2}$ pink grapefruit.
- 25g branflakes with 140ml skimmed milk; 1 medium banana.

LUNCHES

- Sandwich of 2 slices bread filled with 60g peeled prawns and salad; Any individual pot low-fat fruit fromage frais, any flavour.
- 1 white large pitta bread split and filled with 50g hummus and a variety of chopped firm salad items such as cucumber, peppers, celery, onion, tomato. Lettuce and cress can be added if eating straight away.
- 1 × 450ml pack St Michael Tomato and Basil soup sprinkled with 1 rounded tablespoon grated half-fat mozzarella cheese, 1 WeightWatchers soft brown roll or 1 slice bread.
- 1 Boots Shapers tuna and cucumber sandwich; 1 large banana.

EVENING MEALS

- 1 portion Penne Primavera (see recipe page 48).

- 1 portion Sweet and Sour Pork and Noodles (see recipe page 47).
- ½ a 283g can ratatouille heated and mixed with 50g (dry weight) pasta shapes, cooked, and topped with 1 tablespoon grated Parmesan cheese; salad.
- 1 medium rainbow trout (250g), cooked without fat; 125g new or boiled potatoes; 4 tablespoons peas; unlimited greens; horseradish sauce.
- Omelette made with 2 medium eggs cooked in a non-stick pan sprayed with Fry Light, filled with chopped mushrooms; 1 small wholemeal roll; salad; 1 Müller Light 200g pot fruit yogurt.

HEALTHY SNACKS

- 1 rounded tablespoon hummus on 1 dark rye Ryvita.
- 5 dried ready-to-eat apricots plus one apple.
- 40g tzatziki (yogurt and cucumber) with raw carrot or other vegetable plus one Grissini stick.

SWEET TREATS RECORD

	Had	Calories	Running Total
Monday			
Tuesday			
Wednesday			
Thursday			
Friday			
Saturday			
Sunday			
Week Total			1,400 calories

SWEET-TOOTH RECIPES

150 CALORIES OR UNDER

CHOCOLATE PEARS

Serves 4
150 calories and 2.5g fat per portion

4 nice large pears – e.g. William or Conference
Lemon juice
50ml golden syrup
2 level tablespoons cocoa powder
1 × 100ml portion any WeightWatchers icecream

Peel the pears leaving stalks in place, cut off bottoms to make a flat base, brush with lemon juice and put upright in a small saucepan in about 2cm of water. Bring to a simmer, cover and cook gently until tender.

Meanwhile, heat the syrup in a small pan and stir in the cocoa, mixing until you have a smooth sauce. When the pears are cooked, remove from the pan with a slotted spoon and serve with the sauce poured over and a scoop of ice cream on each.

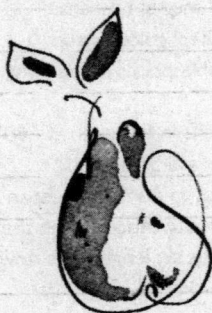

CHOCOLATE AND STRAWBERRY MERINGUES

Serves 4
150 calories and 2.5g fat per portion

Any individual pot chilled chocolate mousse
containing 100 calories or less
4 ready-made meringue nests
100g strawberries
1 level dessertspoon icing sugar
4 good squirts of Anchor aerosol cream, any flavour

Spoon half a chocolate pudding into each of the meringue nests. Slice the strawberries and fill each nest, then dust with icing sugar. Top each with a good squirt of aerosol cream and serve immediately.

NOTE *You could use raspberries or stoned halved cherries in this recipe instead of strawberries.*

BAKED BANANAS WITH CHOCOLATE SAUCE

Serves 4
132 calories and 1g fat per portion

4 medium bananas
50ml golden syrup
2 level tablespoons cocoa powder

Bake the bananas in their skins in the oven at 180°C/350°F/Gas 4 for 20 minutes or until the skins are blackened.

Meanwhile, heat the syrup in a small saucepan and stir in the cocoa powder until you have a smooth sauce. When the bananas are cooked, serve each on a plate, slit lengthways down the top with the sauce poured into the open skin.

BLACK FOREST DESSERT

Serves 4
150 calories and 5g fat per portion

290g can black cherries in juice
1 teaspoon arrowroot powder
1 sachet instant hot chocolate drink
100g 8 per cent fat fromage frais
Any individual pot chilled chocolate mousse
containing 100 calories or less

Drain the cherries, reserving the juice. Heat the juice in a pan with the arrowroot until you have a thickened sauce. In a mug or small heatproof bowl, mix the sachet of hot chocolate with enough boiling water to make a smooth chocolate sauce the consistency of single cream, then mix the sauce into the fromage frais. Dividing the cherries, cherry sauce, fromage frais and mousses evenly between four glass dishes or glasses, make each dessert as follows: spoon half the cherries into the dishes; spoon the fromage frais/chocolate sauce in next, then the chocolate mousse and finally the rest of the cherries topped with the cherry sauce.

CHOCOLATE BROWNIES

Makes 12
120 calories and 4.5g fat each

Fry Light spray
175g McVitie's Go Ahead Caramel Crunch biscuits
75g Rice Krispies
75g half-fat Anchor spread
50ml golden syrup
Any individual pot chilled chocolate mousse
containing 100 calories or less

Spray a square non-stick baking tin with the Fry Light spray. Crush the biscuits between kitchen parchment with a rolling pin and mix with the Rice Krispies. Melt the half-fat spread and syrup in a small pan and mix into the biscuit mixture. Stir in the mousses and mix everything together well, then smooth into the baking tin and allow to set in the refrigerator for a few hours before cutting into 12 pieces.

200 CALORIES OR UNDER

PEAR AND CHOCOLATE HONEY CREAMS

Serves 4
200 calories and 4.5g fat per portion

1 x 400g can pears in juice, drained
2 Halo Honey Malt chocolate bars
100g 8 per cent fat fromage frais
100g half-fat crème fraîche
2 x 200g pots Müller Light vanilla yogurt
1 level tablespoon runny honey

Chop the pears and place in four individual glass dishes or glasses. Chop the Halo bars and spoon half over the pears. Blend together the fromage frais and crème fraîche and spoon a quarter into each dish. Spoon the vanilla yogurt over the top and finish with the rest of the chopped chocolate and a drizzle of honey on each dessert.

COFFEE, TOFFEE AND CHOCOLATE DELIGHTS

Serves 4
175 calories and 7.2g fat per portion

8 sponge fingers
6 tablespoons strong coffee
3 × 150g Shape low-fat toffee yogurts
2 tablespoons Smuckers Light Hot Chocolate Fudge Topping
1 Flake treatsize bar, crumbled

Break the sponge fingers in half and place four halves into four glass dishes or glasses. Pour the coffee evenly over them. Spoon three-quarters of a tub of yogurt into each, heat the topping and drizzle a quarter over each dessert, then sprinkle with the Flake.

ORANGE LIQUEUR FRUIT TRIFLE

Serves 4
200 calories and 3.5g fat per portion

3 trifle sponge cakes, each halved horizontally
1 dessertspoon raspberry jam
175ml orange juice
1 tablespoon orange liqueur, e.g. Grand Marnier
2 small bananas
1 × 290g can Birds low-fat custard
8 squirts aerosol cream

Spread the sponges with the jam, put the halved slices back together again and cut each sponge cake into four. Put three sponge pieces in the base of each of four individual trifle dishes. Mix the orange juice with the liqueur and pour evenly over the sponges. Slice the banana and divide between the dishes, then top immediately with the custard and finish with 2 squirts of aerosol cream each.

PASSION CAKE SLICES

175 calories and 7.5g fat per slice

Fry Light spray
200g plain or wholemeal flour
1 teaspoon baking powder
1 pinch ground cinnamon and ginger
50g half-fat Anchor spread
50g golden caster sugar
1 medium fresh carrot, peeled and grated
60g chopped mixed nuts
4 level tablespoons lemon curd
50ml skimmed milk
1 medium egg
1 × 350g tub 8 per cent fat fromage frais
1 tablespoon icing sugar
1 tablespoon lemon juice

Spray a non-stick oblong baking tin with Fry Light. In a mixing bowl, combine the flour, baking powder and spices. Rub in the half-fat spread, then add the sugar, carrot and mixed nuts. In a small bowl, mix together the lemon curd, skimmed milk and egg until well combined, and add to the flour mixture, stirring well. Spoon into the baking tin and level the surface. Bake at 180°C/350°F/Gas 4 for 30 minutes or until a skewer comes out of the centre clean and the cake looks golden. Turn out and allow to cool.

Meanwhile, make a topping by beating the fromage frais with the icing sugar and lemon juice. Spread over the cake when cool, then cut into 12 slices. The top can be decorated with slices of lemon or walnut halves (20 calories and 2g fat each).

250 CALORIES OR UNDER

QUICK CREAMY BRÛLÉE

Serves 4
240 calories and 13.5g fat per portion

75g mascarpone cheese
200g 8 per cent fat fromage frais
200g low-fat ready-made custard
125g frozen raspberries, blackberries or other soft fruit
4 tablespoons caster sugar

Beat together the mascarpone and the fromage frais, then stir in the custard to combine well.

Meanwhile, heat the fruit in a small pan with $\frac{1}{2}$ tablespoon of the sugar until the juices are just starting to run, and divide between four small heatproof ramekins. Spoon a quarter of the cheese mixture over the top of each of these and level out, then top each with a quarter of the remaining sugar. Grill under a preheated very hot grill to caramelise the sugar. Leave to cool before serving.

CHOCOLATE AND COCONUT CRUNCHIES

Serves 4
247 calories and 14.5g fat per portion

250g tub 8 per cent fat fromage frais
1 sachet low-calorie instant hot chocolate drink
30g desiccated coconut
37g pack Maltesers, crushed
6 gingernut biscuits, lightly crushed

Put the fromage frais in a mixing bowl. Blend the chocolate drink with 30ml boiling water and stir this into the fromage frais. Mix in the coconut and Maltesers. Divide the mixture between four small dishes or glasses and top with the crushed gingernut biscuits.

300 CALORIES OR UNDER

BANOFFEE LAYERS

Serves 4
267 calories and 8g fat per portion

2 bananas
4 individual Shape creamy toffee bio yogurts
1 large Cadbury's Caramel bar
30ml single cream
150ml thick bio yogurt
1 dessertspoon icing sugar
1 Flake treatsize bar

Slice the bananas thinly and arrange in the base of four glass serving dishes or glasses. Spoon half a pot of toffee yogurt into each dish. Melt the Caramel bar in a small pan with the single cream, mix well and divide this mixture between the four dishes. Beat the bio yogurt with the icing sugar and spoon one quarter into each dish. Top with the remaining toffee yogurts and finish by crumbling the Flake and sprinkling it over the top of the desserts.

TIRAMISU

Serves 4
260 calories and 14g fat per portion

12 sponge fingers
50ml Marsala wine
75ml strong coffee
25g fructose
75g mascarpone cheese
200g 8 per cent fat fromage frais
100ml half-fat crème fraîche
1 level tablespoon cocoa powder

Put the sponge fingers in a four-serving trifle bowl. Mix the Marsala, coffee and fructose and pour evenly over the sponge fingers. Beat together the cheese and fromage frais; beat in the crème fraîche and spoon evenly over the fingers. Top with the cocoa powder sieved over.

CALORIE AND FAT GUIDE
to All Your Favourite Sweet-tooth Products

Use this list in conjunction with the instructions for the Sweet-tooth Plan that appear on pages 57–8.

Ices	Calories	Fat (g)
Wall's Magnum White	300	20
Mars (single)	209	12
Nestlé KitKat	218	14.5
Wall's Cornetto, choc'n nut	220	12
Wall's Magnum Classic	295	20

Biscuits and Snack Bars	Calories	Fat (g)
Typical values per biscuit (brands may vary slightly)		
Chocolate digestive	85	4
Chocolate finger	30	1.5
Custard cream	65	3
Digestive	80	4
Gingernut	40	1.3
Jaffa cake	45	1
Rich Tea	40	1.4
Shortcake	65	3.5
Jacob's Club milk	122	6.5
Jordan's Crunchy Bar	155	7.5
Nutri-Grain morning bar, strawberry	140	3
Quaker Harvest Chewy bars	max 100	max 3.7
Mars Tracker, choc chip, individual	196	10.7

Cakes and pastries	Calories	Fat (g)
Mr Kipling Bakewell Slice	137	6.3
Mr Kipling Bramley Apple Pie	230	8.3
Mr Kipling Luxury Mince Pie	250	9.2
Mr Kipling Mini Battenberg	126	2.8
Chocolate eclair, large (average)	260	20
Carrot cake, iced, average 75g slice	300	15
Victoria jam sponge, average 50g slice	200	11
Chocolate fudge cake, average 5g slice	290	15
Rich fruit cake, iced, average 50g slice	180	5
Coffee and walnut sponge, iced, average 50g slice	220	12
Doughnut, jam, average	250	12
Cream or vanilla slice	300	18

Sweets	Calories	Fat (g)
Starburst, 45g	185	3.4
Panda Licorice bar	109	1
Fruit Gums, 1 tube	137	nil
Fruit Pastilles, 1 tube	147	nil
Polo Mints, 1 tube	120	0.3

Chocolates	Calories	Fat (g)
Cadbury's Boost	280	16
Cadbury's Caramel	240	12
Cadbury's Crunchie treatsize	80	3.2
Cadbury's Dairy Milk, standard	255	14.5
Cadbury's Fudge	120	4.5
Fry's Chocolate Cream	215	7
Mars Bar, 65g	295	11.5
Mars Flyte	196	6.6
Mars Milky Way, twin	236	8.6

Nestlé Aero milk, medium	252	14.4
KitKat, 4 finger	244	12.6
Rolos, one tube	250	11
Yorkie, milk, 6 chunk	295	16.5
Toblerone, 32g bar	168	9.2

NOTE *Calorie and fat counts for individual chilled or frozen desserts and yogurts almost always appear on the pack. Any of them can be included in your diet as long as the calorie and fat count falls within your weekly allowance (see pages 57–8).*

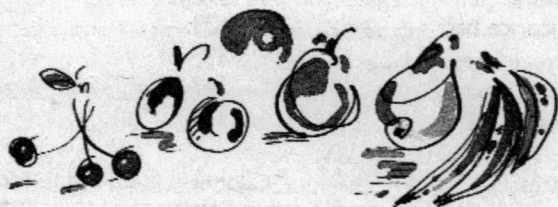

chapter four

the 'e' word

The 3 lb Factor

The two main complaints people have about exercise are that it is boring, and that it doesn't fit in with their lifestyles.

Well, the '3 lb Factor' plan to help you burn off ½ lb of fat a week overcomes both those problems.

In order to burn ½ lb a week, you need to burn off about 1,750 calories over and above those you normally burn. That is an extra 250 calories a day on average.

So I have designed for you a simple chart listing calorie expenditure in 50 activities and the time it will take you to burn off 50 calories, 100 calories or 250 calories doing them.

All you have to do is mix and match your activities every day to a total of 250 and you'll burn that ½ lb of fat. The chart lists the activities in order, starting with those that burn calories quickest, and finishing with the slower ones.

You can pick things you enjoy, that you are capable of doing, and do them in your own time. For instance, to make up a day's calorie burning you could pick:

5 blocks of 50-calorie burn-ups
OR
3 blocks of 50-calorie burn-ups plus one block of 100-calorie burn up

OR
2 blocks of 100-calorie burn-ups plus one 50-calorie block
OR
1 block of 250-calorie burn-up.

It is up to you. However, here are some notes to help you decide:

- Not all the activities listed will provide you with aerobic benefits –
i.e. not all will necessarily improve your heart/lung (cardiovascular)
fitness. For this you need to pick an activity that raises your heart
rate to a training level and maintain it for at least 15 minutes. There
is no real need to get too technical about this – you will know if
you are exercising at a training level if you are slightly 'puffed' while
doing the exercise – i.e. your lungs are working harder and you
maybe can feel your heart beating. You shouldn't feel pain or
exhaustion, but you do need to feel you are working. The items
marked with a * are those that are ideal aerobic activities; and if
you pick them in blocks which provide at least 15 minutes of
training, then your cardiovascular system will get fitter. (Use your
common sense when choosing sports such as football, rugby,
netball and basketball: if you are standing around waiting for the
ball, that isn't aerobic – you need to be moving around briskly
for it to count.)

For the full benefits of exercise as described earlier, it is wise to build
at least three blocks of aerobic exercise into your life every week,
spacing them out evenly through the week.
   All the other activities still burn extra calories, either through short
bursts of activity (which don't count as aerobic) or through using your
muscles for strength.

- If you are very unfit, pick easy types of exercise. I would always go
for walking if you are unsure of your fitness, as you can build up
your fitness safely and gradually. Then when you are fitter, you can

try some of the more demanding activities. If you are unfit and haven't exercised in years, I would have a medical check-up too.

Activities marked with a + are those to save for when you are fitter, or to avoid if you have any medical problems.

• When exercising, wear suitable clothing and don't do vigorous exercise without warming up gently and cooling down afterwards (for example by slowly walking round the room or marching on the spot).

50 Ways to Burn Up Your Daily 250 Calories

* – aerobic + – for fitter people only

Activity	Time taken to burn		
	50 calories (in mins)	100 calories (in mins)	250 calories (in mins)
Squash*+	3½	7	17½
Running*+	4¼	8½	21½
Skipping*	4½	9	22½
Cycling, racing speed*+	4½	9	22½
Cross-country running*+	5	10	25
Stair climbing* (or stair machine)	5	10	25
Healthrider*	5½	11	27½
Swimming, crawl*+	5½	11	27½
Backpacking*+	5½	11	27½
Circuit training	6	12	30
Climbing hills*+	6	12	30
Jogging*+	6¼	12½	31½
Skiing cross-country*+	6¼	12½	31½
Hockey*+	6½	13	32½
Kickboxing+	6½	13	32½
Swimming, breast stroke*	6½	13	32½

Walking, uphill*	6½	13	32½
Horse riding, trot	7	14	35
Netball*	7	14	35
Tennis	7	14	35
Rowing (or machine)	7	14	35
Badminton	7½	15	37½
Cycling, fast*+	7½	15	37½
Dancing, disco*	7½	15	37½
Dancing, line*	7½	15	37½
Digging, heavy	7½	15	37½
Football*+	7½	15	37½
Skiing, downhill*+	7½	15	37½
Mowing, non power-driven*	7½	15	37½
Aerobics class*	8	16	40
Rugby*+	8	16	40
Walking, brisk*	8	16	40
Basketball*	10	20	50
Golf	10	20	50
Gymnastics	10	20	50
Ice skating*	10	20	50
Fencing	10	20	50
Rollerblading*+	10	20	50
Volleyball	10	20	50
Table tennis	11	22	55
Canoeing*	12½	25	62½
Cycling, slow*	12½	25	62½
Polishing	12½	25	62½
Vacuuming	12½	25	62½
Window cleaning	12½	25	62½
Bowls	16½	33	82½
Cricket, batting	16½	33	82½
Cricket, bowling	16½	33	82½
Dancing, ballroom*	16½	33	82½
Horse riding, walk	16½	33	82½